10.15.79

Your Health After 60

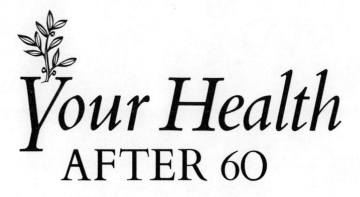

Your Health
AFTER 60

SANDERS-BROWN RESEARCH CENTER ON AGING

M. M. Blacker and D. R. Wekstein, editors

E. P. DUTTON · NEW YORK

For information contact: E. P. Dutton, 2 Park Avenue, New York, N.Y. 10016

Library of Congress Cataloging in Publication Data
Sanders-Brown Research Center on Aging.
    Your health after 60.
    1. Geriatrics.   2. Health.   3. Aging—Physiological aspects.
    I. Blacker, M. M.   II. Wekstein, D. R.   III. Title.
    RC952.S15 1979   613′.0438   79-12080
ISBN: 0-525-93068-X (cloth)
ISBN: 0-525-93082-5 (paper)

Published simultaneously in Canada by Clarke, Irwin & Company Limited, Toronto and Vancouver

Designed by Barbara Huntley

10 9 8 7 6 5 4 3 2 1   First Edition

Contents

Introduction

ONE of the major concerns of the Multidisciplinary
Center of Gerontology at the University of Kentucky
(of which the Sanders-Brown Research Center on
Aging is a part) is the dissemination of information. As
a result of this policy, the Center sponsors a free, public lecture series for the older population of the area.
These lectures (held monthly, during the academic
year) provide the older person with information on a
variety of health-related topics. The lecturer is usually
a faculty member of the Colleges of the A. B. Chandler
Medical Center of the University, and for the past five
years our speakers have given willingly of their time
and expertise.

This book is the outgrowth of the Health Maintenance Lecture Series. It is the Center's belief that an

informed older person is better able to prevent disease, or when that is not possible, is better able to cope with the disease process.

It would be impossible, of course, to cover adequately in a book of this nature all the disease processes from which the older person might suffer; you will notice that we have not covered heart disease or cancer. The omissions were deliberate because we could not discuss, for example, every type of cancer and its treatment. We tried, rather, to touch on topics our lecture audiences were particularly interested in, and in discussing a particular health problem, to provide the reader with some possible means of ameliorating the problem. Naturally, there is no substitute for regular checkups by your family physician; but we are hopeful that this book will give you some insights, lessen some fears, and perhaps suggest to you questions that your physician or other health professional can answer for you.

Demographers predict that by the year 2030 the number of older persons (sixty-five plus) will represent 18 to 22 percent of the population of the United States. That's the future; right now 11 percent of our population is sixty-five plus. We want all of you to stay healthy, happy, and active! We hope this book will contribute in some measure to that goal.

We wish to thank all those who contributed time and energy to our project. Support for this book was provided in part by Grant #90-A-1041 from the Administration on Aging of the Department of Health, Education and Welfare.

David R. Wekstein, Ph.D.
Marcia M. Blacker, M.A.

Lexington, Kentucky
June, 1979

Your Health After 60

1. How to Choose a Physician

J. W. Hollingsworth, M.D.

EVEN healthy people, regardless of their age, need to have plans for how they will seek medical care, when and if it is needed. Beyond age fifty, all of us should have a personal physician as a source of contact with the medical care system, and we should probably have a yearly physical examination. Certainly, once we have developed some chronic illness, we need continuing medical care. Therefore, choosing a physician is a serious business. Before proceeding with advice as to how to make that choice, I think it is wise to consider first what the patient should expect from his or her doctor, and, conversely, what the doctor expects from the patient.

MODERN MEDICAL CARE— REALISTIC EXPECTATIONS

Most of us, when we consider what sort of doctor we want, go back to memories of our childhood when we saw doctors for common infectious ailments that ran their course—illnesses such as measles, mumps, and chicken pox. We remember the doctor as kindly and concerned. Or we conjure up that famous portrait, The Physician, painted by Sir Luke Fildes in the nineteenth century. The painting depicts a sick little child being visited by her physician. He sits by her bed: kind, professional, omnipotent. Yes, we would all like him for our doctor today—*but only if he is medically competent.*

Let's think a little about what Sir Luke's physician might have been doing in that cottage. Tuberculosis was common in England at that time, and perhaps the child was one of the consumptives. The nineteenth-century doctor made his diagnosis only when the disease had progressed so far that it could be detected by that little stethoscope he wore around his neck. He had no skin tests, no X rays, no bacteriologic tests to allow him to make an early diagnosis. Certainly, he had no effective treatment to offer, since the first antibiotic to be effective in tuberculosis was discovered only about thirty years ago. Sir Luke's physician could offer only consolation, and hope nature would help the sick child.

I graduated from medical school about thirty years ago. Many of the diagnostic tests we use today, and almost all of the current drugs, were hardly dreamed of in 1947. Surgical procedures have advanced enormously. Only the wildest dreamer of 1947 would have thought it possible that patients would be living a normal life with a kidney transplanted into them from another individual.

Medicine has changed, within a relatively few years, from an art to a science. There is every reason to think that new advances in science will continue to change medical practice as radically in the next thirty years. Thus, the first and perhaps greatest expectation the patient has of his physician is medical competence.

Somehow, the lay press and television have led the public to believe that physicians must be superhuman. Doctors are expected to be experts on all sorts of social and personal problems, while equally knowledgeable about brain tumors and drug addiction.

These expectations are unrealistic. As Dr. Franz J. Ingelfinger, editor of the *New England Journal of Medicine,* says, "The badges of good medical management are knowledge, honesty, wisdom, and compassion. Honesty and compassion are personal attributes, and wisdom comes from experience, but these qualities are of little real use unless supported by a core of knowledge, an updated acquaintance with medical science."

THE EDUCATION, TRAINING, AND CERTIFICATION OF DOCTORS

When an individual graduates from medical school, he or she must take even further advanced training in order to qualify as a physician. For more than fifty years most states have required at least one year of postgraduate training before granting a physician a license to practice. That year, formerly known as the internship, is now almost universally supplanted by a minimal three-year training program, or residency, in a given specialty. Training may last seven to eight years before the physician is certified in a specialty such as cardiac surgery or neurosurgery.

At the end of the training period or periods, trainees are given a national examination by outstanding members of their specialty discipline. These examinations, called Boards, may consist of oral or written examinations, or observations of the candidate actually at his work. In different years, all of these examination techniques may have been used. When the physician completes the training and passes the examination, he is "boarded" in his discipline, and receives an elaborate scroll that certifies to that fact. This is usually framed and prominently displayed in his office.

The specialty Boards have no role in licensing or in defining what a physician is competent to do. Indeed, licensure carries with it a broad connotation of competence in medicine. I am a Diplomate of the American Board of Internal Medicine, and I practice mostly rheumatology (arthritis). Since the rheumatology Board is a recent creation, I do not have my Board in rheumatology. My state license would allow me to remove your gall bladder or put a catheter into your heart, but my conscience, the wisdom of the hospitals in which I work, and a legitimate fear of a malpractice suit preclude my doing these things to you. I could declare myself a specialist in anything, however, and no one could dispute me until what I did proved harmful to a patient.

Boards do two things: (1) certify to a period of training in a given specialty area, and (2) certify that the physician mastered the material in that specialty to the satisfaction of a group of distinguished members of that discipline. Conversely, absence of Board certification is no sure stigma *against* the competence of a physician. For example, the doctor might have decided against another examination, or might have been an established expert when the particular Board was formed (as in my case with rheumatology). In general, then, being Board-certified insures a minimal quality of competence *at one point in time.* No Board has yet seriously taken upon itself to certify that people have *maintained* their competence.

Since you will be concerned, as a patient selecting a physician, primarily with a broadly trained physician, I think it is worthwhile to review briefly the

Boards in family practice and in internal medicine.

Family practice declared itself a discipline only a few years ago. Most people who have Boards in family practice were general physicians (general practitioners, if you will) when the Boards came into being. By special tests and other requirements, many of those general physicians were certified by the Board of Family Practice without any specific content or time period of training. Since the Board was established, however, many residency programs in family practice have been established, and three years of postmedical school residency are required for new physicians to receive their Board in family practice.

Internal medicine evolved some fifty years ago as a discipline separate from surgery, from those physicians who were known then as *diagnosticians*. Requirements were for three years of postgraduate training in an approved program, and passing an oral examination based on examination of patients. More recently, the oral examination has been supplanted by a written examination. Within internal medicine, subspecialists emerged and developed their own training programs, usually two more years in the subspecialty after three years in general internal medicine. Some subspecialty groups established subspecialty Boards many years ago (cardiology, allergy, gastroenterology, pulmonary diseases). More recently, endocrinology (glands), rheumatology (arthritis), hematology (blood diseases), oncology (cancer), nephrology (kidney disease), and infectious diseases have established subspecialty Boards. So that many legitimate subspecialists in internal medicine may not have their subspecialty Board certificates, but they do have Boards in internal medicine. All, then, have had solid general training in their background.

HOW DOCTORS ORGANIZE
THEIR PRACTICE

No longer do we select "a" doctor; few physicians today practice alone. Some may have primarily a solo practice, but share night and weekend call with other physicians. It is unlikely that any individual physician will be available to you more than half the hours of the week. Thus, you want to think about how his or her practice works, and who is available to you when your doctor is not on call. My situation is an extreme example. As a professor in a university, I take responsibility for my patients but they may see another faculty colleague on occasion. At times they must come to the emergency room of University Hospital to be seen by one of our resident physicians.

A few doctors have a partnership, but more are associated in small groups, perhaps three to six physicians, of the same general background and training. These small groups of internists or family physicians tend to share common facilities and night call, but otherwise each doctor has his own practice. The situation is quite similar to the solo practitioner sharing call, except for greater access to patient records and easier informal in-group consultation. Also, in shared facilities, the patients do get to feel more comfortable with all the physicians in the group and may feel more secure as a result.

Larger groups tend to be multidisciplinary, involving pediatricians, internists with different subspecialties, surgeons, and so forth. The Mayo Clinic is the best known and the biggest of these groups. The advantages are the ready accessibility of facilities and of many kinds of consultants. The disadvantages are that the patient (and his primary physician) are locked into those particular facilities and those particular consultants.

Although most multidisciplinary groups are basic fee-for-service operations, some operate on a prepaid basis. Under that system the patient and his family pay a yearly fee and get as much service as they need. Most of the well-established prepaid groups are closed to older people, but recently the federal government has helped to fund a number of these groups (generally known as Health Maintenance Organizations, HMOs). These usually have open enrollment policies.

There is, in my opinion, no right nor wrong in any of these plans by which doctors organize their practice. In a given locale, with a given set of people, I might prefer one to another. But the patient should consider the system as well as the doctor, and should understand quite definitely who is available when his primary doctor is not on call. So often, catastrophic illness strikes at odd hours.

Finally, severe illness may occur suddenly. If the physician, or his designate, is not immediately available for telephone consultation, call the local ambulance service or rescue squad and take the patient to the nearest hospital that has good emergency coverage. If possible, this hospital should be the one commonly used by your doctor. Once the emergency situation is taken care of, your doctor can be contacted and more definite plans can be made. Remember that in a true emergency, there is probably little that the physician can do in the home; the ambulance squad is usually trained, equipped, and often in direct radio contact with the hospital emergency room.

FITTING THE DOCTOR TO YOUR NEEDS

A given person of any age may be basically healthy and need nothing more than occasional examinations. It is easy, if you are healthy, to make a sloppy choice of a doctor because you figure you really don't need him. However, none of us seems likely to be immortal, and when a doctor is needed you want one who is competent, concerned, and available. Therefore, pick your doctor with the idea that your life, tomorrow, might depend on his skill.

If you have no major health problems, a good general physician is what you need. He can be either a family physician or an internist, depending on your choice. The family physician is likely to cover a broader range of simple ailments. The internist may be somewhat more comfortable with significant chronic diseases of older people. Both should be prepared to do a baseline examination, and to take responsibility for your health. Either one may have to refer you periodically to other specialists for episodes of care (for example, an illness requiring surgery), but should continue as your basic or primary doctor.

You may already have a significant chronic illness, or may develop one while under the care of your primary physician. In those circumstances, you or your doctor may decide that a medical subspecialist is preferable. Diseases such as diabetes, angina pectoris, or rheumatoid arthritis can be handled by a family physician, a general internist, or a medical subspecialist. However, the patient should feel that the doctor knows enough about the disease, and, conversely, the doctor should feel comfortable about taking the responsibility.

Often, in older people, medical care boils down to a continuing battle with some specific chronic disease. In that case, the patient is likely to gravitate to the medical subspecialist if the option is locally available. This is not always done, however. For example, one family physician I know is quite interested and competent in rheumatoid arthritis, and I would hardly advise a patient with that disease to leave his care.

In other older people, the medical problem may not be a single major disease, but several bothersome problems that require continuing care—for example (as above) mild diabetes, rare episodes of angina pectoris, and mild rheumatoid arthritis. In those circumstances a family physician or general internist might be preferable to a number of subspecialists.

HOW CAN I TELL IF MY DOCTOR IS COMPETENT?

Unfortunately, judging the quality of medical practice is difficult for other doctors as well as for patients. Also, all doctors make mistakes. All of us, on occasion, fall short of the human qualities that a patient needs from us.

There are some *very* general guidelines: (1) you, as the patient, should feel that you understand what is being done and why; (2) excessive or highly limited use of laboratory tests or of consultants are both somewhat suspicious; (3) if your complaints are getting worse, and there is no explanation or attempt to find an answer, your doctor may be beyond his competence or may be too distracted to really give you proper care; and (4) you may feel you are getting too many medications, without a good explanation of their anticipated action.

Some people feel that competency can be judged by what occurs during the annual checkup. In my judgment, a patient can spend anywhere from $20 to $2,000 and still not have an adequate examination. Doctors honestly differ as to what should constitute a "checkup." There are a few standard tests: Blood pressure should be checked, and the heart examined. In older men, a rectal examination should be done to feel the prostate gland for tumors. In women, examination of the breasts and vagina is mandatory. Smokers should have an annual chest X ray.

HOW DO I CHANGE DOCTORS?

Too often, a patient will stay with his doctor long after he has lost confidence in the doctor, or he may simply stay away from needed medical care to avoid making a change. Older patients seem to find it particularly difficult to change doctors, a feeling that probably goes back to those earlier and simpler days when medicine was primarily an art. When all a doctor had to offer was his personality, a change was an affront, particularly in a small town with only two or three doctors. Times have changed, and any good doctor should respect the wish of a patient to seek care elsewhere. If the doctor objects, you probably really *need* another doctor.

Today there is no need for any formal notification that you are changing doctors, unless a transfer of records is required. In the latter circumstance, you are almost invariably seeing the doctor regularly and somehow are dissatisfied; if so, politely phone him and tell him you want your records transferred, and to whom.

Although changing physicians is usually a rela-

2. Medicines: Miracle and Menace

Robert Straus, Ph.D.

MODERN medicines have contributed greatly to extending the duration of human life and to improving the quality of life of older people. Without the miracles of medicine, many of us would have succumbed to disease or injury at an earlier age. Many older people are active, productive, and relatively comfortable only because the medicines they take help compensate for or repress the effects of disabling diseases. Our good past experience with medicines tends to support a far-reaching faith in the power of medications and other drugs to prevent or cure disease or provide relief from anxiety, pain, or discomfort. We are supported in this unquestioning faith by the advertising of drug manufacturers and distributors. As a result, today patients and physicians alike have developed a deep-seated sense of dependence on drugs.

Evidence of the use of medicines and other drugs that modify our body functions can be traced far back to early primitive societies. Throughout history, virtually all human societies have had drugs that they have associated with the preservation of life. As with other behaviors that have persisted through time, the widespread and persistent uses of drugs and other substances have been perceived as meeting basic needs through recognizable functions or desired effects. Because of the many benefits they offer as painkillers, mood modifiers, or infection fighters, many people tend to think of medicines only in terms of their desired effects or functions.

Unfortunately, all of the medicines and other chemicals that people use are capable of producing a wide range of effects in the human body. While some of these are good, others can be harmful. For example, aspirin can relieve pain, combat inflammation, and reduce fever, but it can also cause stomach discomfort or excessive bleeding. Coffee can help us wake up and stay alert but it can also interfere with our sleep. Alcohol can relieve tension and provide a sense of well-being; it can also cause intoxication and lead to addiction. Drugs that combat excessive anxiety or the "discomfort of colds" can also produce drowsiness or disorientation. This list could go on and on. Depending on how they are used, all drugs have a potential for harm as well as good. The same can be said for drug-like substances such as sugar and salt.

The goal to which we aspire in using drugs of any

kind is to maximize their desired effects or functions and to minimize their adverse affects or dysfunctions. This goal becomes increasingly important as people get older. This is because, with aging, there tend to be more conditions that can benefit from medicines; more medicines are used; and there are significant changes in the processes by which our bodies absorb, metabolize, store, and excrete medicines. Therefore, as people get older, they encounter more potential liabilities and dangers from medicine misuse at the same time that the perceived need for medicines and their potential benefits looms larger.

OLDER PEOPLE USE MORE MEDICINES

It has been reported that people over sixty-five years of age in the United States, while comprising about 10 percent of the population, consume 25 percent of all prescription drugs. This is in part because of the increased prevalence, in older people, of heart and kidney diseases, high blood pressure, diabetes, cancer, arthritis, and other degenerative diseases. While drugs do not prevent or reverse these conditions, they do help the body compensate for deficiencies or provide relief from disabling inflammation or pain. The National Center for Health Statistics has reported that in 1975 the out-of-pocket costs of prescription medicines averaged $31.00 for all noninstitutionalized persons in the United States, but for those who were age sixty-five and older this cost was $76.00. Persons in that age bracket bought on the average more than twice as many prescriptions than the population as a whole, and older people paid significantly more for each prescription. The National Council on Aging has reported that 20 percent of the out-of-pocket expenditures of the elderly goes for drugs.

In a Washington, D.C., study of 5,600 people over age sixty, more than half were using from two to four prescription drugs daily. Drugs for cardiovascular problems or arthritis and tranquilizers accounted for half of all the prescription drugs taken. For a third of these older people the prescription drugs they were taking were seen as essential in order to permit them to perform their daily tasks. In the same population, more than two-thirds were regularly using over-the-counter drugs; half of these were internal analgesics such as aspirin. One-half of the group studied were combining prescription drugs with nonprescription drugs and alcohol.

Numerous recent studies have identified an alarming amount of serious illnesses caused by the misuse of medicines. It has been estimated that 3 to 5 percent of all hospital admissions in the United States are for the treatment of adverse drug reactions or drug-induced diseases. The drugs contributing to such problems include both prescribed and over-the-counter remedies. Often multiple drug use is involved. Common diseases that result from drug misuse can involve all major body organs and can include tumors, excessive bleeding, and chemical imbalance. Because elderly people tend to take more drugs and often use numerous drugs simultaneously, the chances of suffering from drug misuse are enhanced at the same time that their vulnerability to illness in general is increasing. It has also been found that from 15 to 30 percent of hospitalized patients experience one or more adverse reactions from the medicines they are taking during their hospitalization. Again, older people, who tend to have more illnesses and are often receiving several different medicines at the same time, are clearly the most vulnerable.

Although the problems of medicine misuse are not new, we have become more aware of them in recent years. This is partly because of the increasing number and complexity of available drugs. Also, as the potential benefits of drugs have grown, the potential problems that can occur if they are not properly used have also increased.

Because our awareness and concern about these problems has been fairly recent, we still have relatively little research directly aimed at preventing or reducing the problems of medicine misuse. Yet, there are some definite things that we know and some suggestions we can make about how to avoid or minimize the adverse effects of medicines.

ALL PEOPLE ARE UNIQUE

One of the major factors that is now recognized as basic to safe medicine use is recognition of the fundamental individuality of human beings. Only when compared with other species of life are human beings all "alike." When compared with each other, we all have many unique characteristics, including not only external factors such as facial appearance and finger-prints, but also basic biological factors such as our cells and the immune mechanisms and chemistry of our bodies. These variabilities are almost endless and they are quite significant to the different ways in which our bodies may respond to medicines or any other substances that we use. Some people seem able to go through life eating anything and everything they want without ever gaining too much weight. Many people, however, struggle constantly with a weight problem. Some people experience an effect from one drink that others won't experience unless they have two or three. We are now learning that there are comparable differences in the effects that people experience from medicines. Some people need fairly large amounts of a given drug in order to achieve desired effects and may hardly notice undesired effects. Others will get a desired effect from small amounts but will encounter adverse effects if they take more than they need for the desired effect. Some people can't tolerate drugs that other people find beneficial. The way our bodies absorb, break down, utilize, and eliminate all substances—whether food or drug—depends on how our body systems (liver, kidney, stomach, intestines, and blood vessels) function; and, although we are all relatively similar as human beings, no two people have systems that function in exactly the same way.

Not only do we differ from one another in our responses to medicines and other substances, but all of us also vary within ourselves. The impact we experience from a particular drug may depend on such factors as fatigue, illness, mood, what we have recently eaten, and the time of day when the drug is taken. Numerous studies of human behavior around the twenty-four-hour period of day and night indicate that many of our basic body functions fluctuate on a cyclical basis. These include body temperature, heart rate, blood pressure, and some of the metabolic processes that are central to how we respond to drugs. Thus, for some people, the desired balance between beneficial and adverse effects may depend on varying the dose at different times rather than taking a standard dose every few hours.

THE IMPORTANCE OF TIME

Time is a crucial factor in the management of medicines in many ways. It is important to consider how long it takes a particular substance to break down so that it can be absorbed, how long it takes the body to distribute, metabolize or utilize, and eventually excrete the substance. These variations are often crucial in determining the effects of a drug and the degree of its beneficial or undesirable impact. Quite logically, these biological responses will depend on the time intervals between doses, the amount of a drug used at a time, and the form in which the drug is taken.

Time orientation is another factor that is significant in the use of medicine. This is the sense of importance we attach to events in terms of past, present, or future. Some of the medicines we use, such as those for hypertension, are taken in order to prevent future problems by people who actually don't feel sick. Whenever drugs are being used for prevention, the motivation for taking such drugs depends on the user's having a sense of the future.

Time orientation can also mean the sense of importance we attach to being "on time" or to regulating our lives according to a time schedule. People for whom timeliness does not have much value will have difficulty adhering to a time schedule for taking medications and may well get into difficulty if the time factor is indeed crucial to the effective or safe use of drugs.

Several time cycles are also important. We have already mentioned the significance of the daily cycle. In women, the menstrual cycle includes hormonal and other changes in body chemistry and function that are relevant to the utilization of certain medicines and food substances. Annual seasonal cycles that alter environmental factors, such as temperature or humidity and the periods of light and darkness, can be relevant. Perhaps most significant of all is the life cycle.

DRUGS AND THE LIFE CYCLE

Until quite recently, studies of human development and behavior have placed an overwhelming emphasis on the importance and significance of infancy and early childhood. Once maximum physical growth and the social status of adulthood had been achieved, it was popularly assumed that characteristics like intelligence, biological structure and function, and the clustering of personal traits that we call personality became relatively fixed. In many ways we have tended to have one set of assumptions, responses, customs, and expectations for children and another for adults. Although we have recognized that children go through developmental stages with different needs and capacities, we have tended to ignore the obvious broad range of differences that exist among adults as well as the many significant changes that individual adults experience as they progress through the life cycle.

Our differing treatment of children and adults is clearly demonstrated by our customs and laws regarding the use of substances such as alcohol, tobacco, and caffeine. It is also seen in our practices and assumptions regarding the prescribing and use of medicines. As far as medicine taking is concerned, we seem to assume that all adults are equal, irrespective of sex, size, body weight, activities, health, disabilities, or age.

On an individual basis, most people recognize that many of their needs, capacities, and sensitivities change as they get older. Take coffee or other forms of caffeine, for example. Many people realize, at some time in their thirties or forties or fifties, that they are becoming more sensitive to caffeine, particularly as it affects their ability to sleep. They may decide not to drink coffee with their evening meal or even to abstain from caffeine after the middle of the day. Similarly, some individuals in their fifties or later begin to recognize that the amount of alcohol to which they have been accustomed is beginning to produce more noticeable and sometimes unwelcome effects. Most aging people find that they need to eat less food or less of certain kinds of food if they are to avoid gaining weight or feeling uncomfortable.

Yet, despite the fact that as individuals we tend to recognize these changes, our social customs reflect the assumption that all adults are the same. Thus, in social gatherings or public places where food and drinks are served, the amounts normally offered are geared to the comfortable capacities of people who can eat or drink relatively large amounts. We are caught in a silly game of amenities in which the good host and hostess will eat and drink in company with the guest who takes the most, and the good guest will show appreciation by accepting all that is offered. In public restaurants, perhaps because we must pay for large portions regardless of what we want or need, we often feel obliged to clean our plates.

As noted, similar attitudes govern medicine prescribing practices and self-medication. Despite our knowledge about differences between people and variations within individuals that affect the way we respond to drugs, most medicines are prescribed in terms of normal adult doses, with no concern for age. The directions that drug manufacturers provide physicians for prescription medicines and the directions that accompany nonprescription medicines almost invariably indicate different dose levels for children and adults but say nothing about age or other differences among adults. Yet, for some people, these differences can be very significant.

THE BODY-DRUG RELATIONSHIP WITH AGING. In discussing the kinds of change in response to drugs that can occur as people get older, it is important to stress that for some people these changes are hardly noticeable, for others they are moderate, and for some they are considerable. The same is true of other cyclical changes. For example, some women are hardly aware of their menstrual periods; others are incapacitated.

The major processes that are involved in determining the effect we experience from drugs are absorption, metabolism, and excretion. Absorption may be directly into the blood when medicines are injected or indirectly through the stomach and intestines when they are taken by mouth. Metabolism involves changes that occur as the body uses or reacts to the drug. Excretion is the process by which unused or waste products of the drug are eliminated from the body. With aging, changes can occur that affect the rates of all these processes and they can occur in either direction, depending on the drug. Generally, the slower the absorption, and the more rapid the metabolism and the excretion, the less effect a drug may have, while rapid absorption and slow metabolism and excretion will increase the effect. But, unfortunately, drugs and people don't react to each other this simply. Since drugs have multiple effects, some of the effects can be enhanced by the same processes that decrease other effects. Since people have unique and changeable body chemistries, their sensitivities to certain effects of certain drugs can change independent of rates of absorption, metabolism, or excretion.

It is important to recognize that as people get older, their responses to certain drugs can change. For people who have been taking a particular drug for many years, this means that a dose level that is effective and relatively nontoxic during one period of their life may become excessive and toxic as they get older—or the reverse may occur.

This picture is further complicated by the fact that as people get older they tend to have multiple health problems for which medications are used. Among the most significant factors in changing the functions and dysfunctions of the medicines we use are the other drugs we are using at the same time. All drugs can alter both the chemistry and function of our body. Essentially, that's why we use them. When people are taking many drugs, the interactions between these drugs can produce several kinds of undesirable effects.

First, one drug can block or intefere with the effectiveness of another. People using any of the tetracycline antibiotics should be advised not to take these within a couple of hours of using a milk product or one of the common antacid medicines. If they do mix these substances, they will block the absorption and reduce the antibiotic effect of the tetracycline.

Second, one drug can offset or balance out the desired effect of another. People who use sedative drugs to combat insomnia may cancel out the effect if they also use stimulant drugs or drink a great deal of coffee.

Third, one drug can duplicate the impact of another so that the net effect is more than desired. Someone using an anticoagulant or "blood-thinning" drug should never use aspirin because aspirin, in addition to relieving pain, fever, and inflammation, is also an anticoagulant. The combination of aspirin and other anticoagulants could cause dangerously excessive bleeding.

Fourth, drugs can interact so that one drug reverses the balance between the functions and the dysfunctions of another drug. Aspirin, taken occasionally and in moderation, seems safe for most people and remarkably effective in producing several desired functions, although there is a risk that it will cause undesired stomach discomfort and a slight risk that it will cause dangerous bleeding. However, when aspirin is taken along with alcohol, especially if both drugs are taken in fairly large amounts, the combination greatly increases the probability of an adverse or dangerous effect from aspirin.

Fifth, many drugs interact so that the net effect is greater than the sum of the parts. Often this so-called "synergistic" process is sought intentionally as when aspirin and codeine are prescribed in combination to produce a more effective relief from pain. But often people quite innocently use drugs that can be synergistic in a dangerous way. Valium, the popular anti-anxiety drug, is prescribed about sixty million times a year in the United States. Alcohol is used regularly by more than one hundred million people. Both Valium and alcohol can produce drowsiness and can depress brain function including motor responses and thought processes. Valium and alcohol, in most people, interact to enhance the combined effect. Thus, anyone using a generally "safe and effective" amount of Valium at the same time that they are consuming a generally "safe and effective" amount of alcohol can experience a dangerous and toxic combined result. Similarly, such "one plus one equals three" results can occur when the usually relatively "safe" antihistamines that some twenty to thirty-five million people are taking in cold remedies, allergy medicines, or non-prescription sleeping pills are combined with Valium or other anti-anxiety drugs or with alcohol.

OTHER EXAMPLES OF MEDICINE MISUSE. The problems that people experience in using medicines as they
get older are by no means restricted to such matters as
taking more of a drug than they need, experiencing
more bad than good effects from a drug, or encountering complications from the interaction of several
drugs that are being used at the same time. Many
older people are living on reduced incomes and can't
afford to buy the medicines they need. Some may try
to stretch out their supply and take less than they
need. Others have no transportation or no one to help
in getting their prescriptions filled. Many older people
report serious problems in trying to cope with child-
proof medicine containers that respond more easily to
the digital dexterity of a seven-year-old than to the ar-
thritic manipulations of people past fifty. Frequently,
patients, regardless of age, have difficulty hearing or
understanding the directions that their physicians give
them regarding the proper way to use a drug. This is a
problem because such directions are usually given
only once, often hurriedly, and in settings that are not
conducive to listening or hearing. Often, the directions
are incomplete and fail to anticipate the special circumstances under which individuals have to work out
their drug-using practices. When people are using several medications simultaneously, each of which has its
own set of precautions, dosage, and frequency of use,
the opportunities and probabilities for confusion increase all the more. Most people, old and young alike,
keep their medicines in bathrooms or kitchens where

exposure to steam and moisture may cause deterioration and chemical change in some drugs. Some people keep medicines in open dishes where they are easy to get at but exposed to spoilage from air, light, or dampness. Most people hoard unused medicines far beyond the time when these can be safely taken. Many people exchange medicines with family or friends or self-medicate without even knowing what they are taking.

THE IMPORTANCE OF COMMUNICATION ABOUT MEDICINES

For nonprescription medicines, most people rely heavily on advertising and on the directions that come with their drugs. Most directions suggest only normal adult dosages and do not even imply that many people may need less, especially as they get older. Most advertisements emphasize the "strength" and the "power" of the product; often they imply that if two are good, four are better. Rarely are there precautions against overdosage, and almost never are there warnings against drug interactions that should be avoided. Technically, such information is provided in accordance with law on inserts that accompany each package. In reality, the tiny print and technical language of package inserts tend to obscure the warnings. Most prescription medicines carry even less information than nonprescription drugs; no more, usually, than can be typed on a tiny label. Many of the problems of drug misuse lie in faulty communications, and at least some of the solutions depend on the communicators. These include the pharmaceutical industry, prescribers, pharmacists, and patients. All can play a part.

The manufacturers of drugs can clearly improve the level of truth and clarity they provide in advertising, promoting, and labeling their products. Prescribers of drugs can improve their own level of knowledge abut the products they prescribe and the patients for whom they are prescribing. They can have better knowledge about adverse effects, changes in metabolism with aging, and potential problems of drug interaction. They should seek full histories of patients' past experiences with medications and other drug substances and they should be sure that patients know what medications they are taking in the present and for what reason. They should seek to learn how patients normally respond to various types of drugs, and should provide opportunities for monitoring the experiences of their patients with the medications that they are prescribing. Prescribers should also take time to explain carefully to each patient, for each medication, the name, appearance, purposes, dosage, and possible adverse signs. They should determine whether the patient is capable of understanding and carrying out their instructions. All verbal instructions should be accompanied by written directions that the patient can take, keep, and refer to.

Modern pharmacists, who receive extensive training in pharmacology and therapeutics can often help the physician and the patient in many ways beyond simply filling the prescription. Some pharmacists now assist by obtaining medicine-use histories from patients for physicians and by supplementing the physician's limited time with each patient by repeating the physician's instructions. Pharmacists can report back to physicians information or questions about adverse effects or drug interactions. Many pharmacists are also able to provide patients with general instructions and warnings that go beyond the limited information on the prescription label.

Patients can play the most important role of all in improving communication about medicines and in safeguarding their own use of medicines. They can be sure that they provide physicians (or other prescribers such as dentists) with full information about all medicines or drug-like substances that they are using and about any unpleasant responses they have had to medicines in the past. They can be sure that they understand what physicians tell them about each medication that is prescribed. What is it? What is it for? How should it help? When, how often, in what amounts should it be taken? Should it be used before, during, or after meals? What possible adverse effects might occur? What foods or other substances should *not* be used with the medicine? How should it be stored? If any of the questions are not covered by the physician or are not understood, the patient should ask again. The patient should request instructions in writing from the physician, or if the physician prefers, from the pharmacist. If questions remain after the prescription is filled, the patient should not hesitate to call the physician, or ask the pharmacist, or request that the pharmacist call the physician. If unanticipated or unpleasant effects from the drug are experienced, the patient should inform the physician immediately.

The miracles of modern medicine have led us to have great expectations. We assume that whenever we are given or elect to take medicine it will be good for us. But because of our great faith in medicines, we often tend to accept too much of the "bitter" with the "sweet." Most modern medicines have potential for producing both good and bad effects. The effect that a particular patient will experience with a particular drug depends on matching the drug with the patient in a number of ways. Matching medicines with patients requires full and clear communication involving manufacturers, physicians, pharmacists, and patients. Since patients are in the position to gain or lose the most from the medicines they use, they should never hesitate to ask questions, and to insist on answers they can understand.

2072402

3. Arthritis and Bone Problems

J. W. Hollingsworth, M.D.

To understand some of the bone problems in older people, we must understand that bone is not the concrete-looking structure it seems. In the living person, bone is composed of a groundwork of protein on which various minerals such as calcium, phosphorus, and sodium are deposited to form a strong skeletal structure. The protein matrix, like other body proteins, is constantly being renewed from amino acids in the blood.

As we age, all body proteins change in their chemical characteristics and, consequently, in their functional aspects. Changes in the eye, discussed elsewhere in this book, are excellent examples. Another example of protein change occurs in skin. Loss of elastic proteins causes wrinkling and thinning, producing the fine parchment-like skin we see in the very old. Similar changes occur in the matrix of bone.

The minerals of bone, also, are not static. Calcium,

sodium, and phosphorus are being constantly inter-
changed between blood and bone. Indeed, bone is a
rich reservoir of these elements, a reservoir that the
body calls upon when in need. The ability of the bone
matrix (protein) to hold onto minerals and to organize
them into highly complex bone becomes less efficient
with age. In addition, bone must get its minerals (calcium in particular) from the diet, and intestinal absorption of calcium depends upon vitamin D and
complex hormonal interactions. Frequently, older
people do not have a proper diet and may lack necessary vitamin D.

THINNING OF BONE (OSTEOPOROSIS)
WITH AGE

As we grow older, the net result of changes in bone
matrix is a thinning of bone. Men have thicker bones
than do women, and therefore women's bones get
dangerously thin more frequently and earlier in life.
Blacks, men and women, have thicker bones than their
Caucasian counterparts.

Thinning of bone can be detected primarily by X
rays, which show less dense bone than normal. Special
X-ray techniques have been developed to actually
measure bone density so that the effects of treatments
can be assessed, but clinically, we remain unaware of
osteoporosis until a bone actually breaks. There is,
however, remarkably good correlation between osteoporosis and thin skin. Glistening tendons showing

through the skin on the back of the hand probably indicate significant osteoporosis.

FRACTURES OF BONES

The result of osteoporosis is fractures of bones, which may occur spontaneously; the vertebrae of the low back are common sites of such breaks. Other bones also fracture spontaneously, but less frequently.

Fractures often occur after only slight injury. The incidence of fractures of the wrist and of the hip goes up strikingly beyond age sixty. Indeed, broken hips have become a dreaded disease of older age because complications from these fractures are a significant cause of death.

RETARDATION AND TREATMENT
OF OSTEOPOROSIS

Retarding the progress of osteoporosis has not yet proven medically feasible, but understanding how osteoporosis works suggests some sensible advice. You should drink two or three glasses of milk daily because milk has protein, calcium, and vitamin D. Skim milk, since it has the necessary vitamins without the fat, is fine for those people who need to watch their weight. Vitamin D in large therapeutic doses (50,000 units/day) has been recommended in the past, but is potentially harmful. A well-balanced diet with milk seems best. Of course, foods containing milk, such as cheese and ice cream, are also acceptable sources of this vitamin and these minerals.

Moderate exercise helps increase bone density. Since inactivity leads to rapid and dramatic osteoporosis, it seems reasonable that moderate activities such as walking and swimming would help retard osteoporosis.

Sex hormones play a role in osteoporosis. Women who have their ovaries removed or who have spontaneous menopause find their osteoporosis speeded up; estrogen hormone treatment definitely retards the process. Estrogens have other effects, desirable and undesirable. Recently there has been much discussion about estrogen causing cancer of the breast and uterus. Using estrogen therapy is, therefore, a difficult decision that should be made by patient and physician in consultation.

Treatment, once a fracture of a vertebra or some other bone has occurred, is also a subject of controversy. Some physicians employ hormones, some prescribe only calcium and additional vitamin D, and some prescribe fluoride in addition to calcium. Other good physicians do little, because the benefits of any of these treatments have yet to be proved and the progression of osteoporosis is generally slow.

AGING OF JOINTS AND OSTEOARTHRITIS

All of us who have separated the long leg from the short leg on a chicken know a bit about the normal

anatomy of a joint. First, there are strong, tough ligaments of protein connective tissue that support the
joint; in the chicken's leg they are hard to cut through.
Once separated, the ends of the bones are glistening
and smooth to touch. Those ends are not bone, but articular cartilage, a highly specialized tissue that cush-
ions against weight and injury. The slimy fluid in the
joint is a remarkable lubricant that allows bones and
ligaments to slide over each other smoothly. Hydraulic
engineers envy the efficiency of this fluid!

As we age, pressures on our joints cause a slow and
progressive remolding of those articular surfaces related to the use of our joints and to weight-bearing.
Something happens so that cartilage cells begin to deteriorate and produce scars and fissures in that smooth
cartilage surface. Cells begin to multiply in an attempt
to repair the damage. As the process expands and extends, bone cells begin to proliferate and form extra
bony spurs and ridges where bone and cartilage unite.
In the joint, then, we see by X-ray examination less
cartilage and the formation of new bone in irregular
places and shapes. We call this formation *osteoarthritis*.

Osteoarthritis is a normal part of aging, and most
older people have some joint discomfort. The knees,
hips, and the spine, which bear most of the weight, are
common scources of complaint. Fingers take enormous
pressure even with "normal" use. There is a hereditary
factor, more pronounced in women, in the gnarled
bumpy fingers of old age. In women, those changes

often begin at menopause. However, in nine out of ten women, osteoarthritic fingers are no more than a cosmetic nuisance, and of no real medical concern.

Osteoarthritis becomes severe in only a few patients, and then it usually predominates in one or two joints, primarily the hips and knees. It seems probable that those joints that are rapidly destroyed by osteoarthritis were damaged by an earlier injury or by some other disease such as minimal dislocation of a hip in infancy.

PREVENTION AND TREATMENT OF OSTEOARTHRITIS

Since so much of osteoarthritis really involves cartilage, it seems likely that medical science may eventually be able to define genetic differences in cartilage, or may produce drugs that improve the health of cartilage. However, that is in the future.

At present we know that an injury (trauma) may cause us to develop osteoarthritis. Most trauma, however, occurs in our youth and is not amenable to prevention. We can, however, avoid exercises that make our knees or hips hurt worse. That sign—increased pain after activity—indicates that we are overdoing on exercise. We can control our weight since each pound adds greatly to the pressure on our weight-bearing joints.

Once osteoarthritis is advanced in a given joint,

surgery may be advisable. One of the truly great advances in medicine is the total hip joint replacement,
made possible by modern technology. Many older
people look on the operation as a miracle since it gives
them normal mobility and freedom from pain.

FIBROCARTILAGE, AND NECK AND BACK PROBLEMS

In addition to the smooth, glistening cartilage that
caps our long bones, there is another tougher material,
fibrocartilage, that helps keep bones in place and
serves as a pad for the bones of our spine. The wedges
of cartilage that help support the sides of our knees,
and are the subject of the "torn cartilage" of the young
athlete, are good examples. The "discs" of the spine
are the tough plates or pads that separate our vertebrae. These structures of fibrocartilage, about a quar-
ter inch in height, allow our spine remarkable mobility
and the ability to withstand stress without damaging
the delicate spinal cord that lies within our vertebrae.
All the nerves of the body leave the spinal cord
through holes in the vertebrae, to connect with our
skin and muscles and blood vessels.

The makeup of our spine—bones, ligaments, and
discs—is indeed a miracle of creation that allows man
(uniquely among mammals) to maintain a totally
erect posture. But this wonderful structure, and particularly the discs between vertebrae, undergoes the rav-
ages of time and trauma like all of our skeleton. The

most evident result of deterioration of our spinal discs is the loss of height as we grow older. Many normal people lose an inch or two of height as the discs flatten with age.

As discs deteriorate, accompanying osteoarthritic changes affect the vertebrae, resulting in a loss of motion. Many older people have trouble moving their neck easily from side to side, and tend to move their entire body rather than twist their neck as they look from side to side. Usually there is some pain or at least mild discomfort when such a motion is attempted.

Similar changes occur in the vertebrae of the low back, so that we bend and twist in less agile and more uncomfortable ways. These changes are less frequent in our midspine area, which moves less than the neck or low back because those vertebrae form attachments to the ribs and are part of a semirigid chest cage.

Major symptoms occur when a deteriorating disc ruptures. The inner core of the disc is a gel-like spongy material, which, when the disc suddenly deteriorates, perhaps presses outward toward one or more of the large nerves leaving the spinal canal. When this occurs in the low back, the common symptom of *sciatica* results. The nerves that run down the buttocks and back of the legs are pressed or irritated, causing pain running down the legs from the buttocks area. If pressure is more severe, loss of nerve sensation of the skin or part of the leg may result, and more important, there may be loss of motion of the foot or leg as nerves supplying muscles are damaged. In rare cases a ruptured disc may even compress the spinal nerves that supply the bladder, and cause paralysis of this organ. In the neck, the same process may compress a nerve to the shoulder, arm, and/or hand with resulting pain, loss of sensation, or loss of motion.

Treatment of disc disease and/or spinal osteoarthritis depends on the severity of the disability. Obviously, acute bladder paralysis or acute inability to move a foot may require emergency surgery. We now do far less surgery for sciatica since we have learned that many acute episodes subside with rest alone. Sometimes, however, surgery is essential. If the problem is in the neck, a collar or brace may help, but surgery is occasionally required. Aspirin and other drugs may help relieve pain.

The best way to prevent spine disease is to maintain life-long good posture. Mild back exercises may help provide better muscle tone and support, but these exercises should be under supervision of a physician or physical therapist. Low-back problems often arise from improper lifting. Lift from a bent-knee position, rather than pulling up directly with the low back. This motion allows the legs and not the back to support the lifting.

ON THE VIRTUES OF THE CANE

Man's first tool, undoubtedly, was a stick used for probing, defense, and support. Somehow, older people resent going about with a cane or walking stick, but many of the falls that prove so devastating could probably be prevented with the added stability offered by a cane. A cane can take some weight off a painful hip or knee or back.

The changes in bone or cartilage we have discussed contribute to loss of agility with aging. In addition, muscles are less strong, nerve reflexes are slowed, and nerve sensation decreases. Older people are prone to minor episodes of dizziness and light-headedness. All of these factors add to the increased likelihood of falling, and are cogent reasons to use a cane. Frankly, I think the older person looks dignified with a cane, and often helpless and doddery when walking unaided.

It is important to remember that osteoporosis can be retarded and treated; proper attention to diet and moderate exercise both contribute to the treatment. Osteoarthritis is a normal part of aging, and while it may cause some disfigurement, it is not life-threatening and generally leads to only minimal discomfort which can be alleviated by not overdoing exercise and by controlling weight. The natural process of aging produces a variety of changes in our bodies; fortunately, for most of us, our minds remain active and agile. Using our minds to keep occupied, involved, and happy is the best medicine!

4. Dental Health

Charles W. Ellinger, M.Sc., D.D.S.
Jerry L. Stovall, D.M.D.
John W. Unger, D.D.S.
John A. Thompson, D.M.D.

WITH age, many changes occur throughout the body. In the mouth these changes include reduction in saliva, loss of supporting bone, decrease in the elasticity of tissue, reduction in the thickness of the tissue that covers the ridges, and in many instances a loss of muscle tone, power, and coordination.

Many people in their sixties have already lost or will shortly be losing their teeth. Fortunately, some individuals keep their teeth a lifetime. Whichever category you fit in, it is important to practice regular oral hygiene and to have regular dental examinations by your family dentist.

RADIOGRAPHS (X Rays)

Are X rays necessary? Yes, if the dentist is going to diagnose what lies underneath the visible tissue. When the dentist looks in your mouth, he is able to see only the crown portion of the teeth; in patients without teeth, he sees only the soft tissue. X rays allow the dentist to view the roots of teeth and the bone structure. In addition, the dentist is able to detect tooth decay that exists between the teeth, although this type of tooth decay may not be detectable until the decay is well along and by that time there is danger of tooth loss.

Will X rays cause harm? It can be safely said that the amount of radiation caused by dental radiographs when used properly will not harm the individual.

SPECIALTIES OF DENTISTRY

Most individuals start dental treatment with a general dentist. The general dentist is trained to perform most dental procedures that are necessary in the treatment of the patient. However, certain procedures may be beyond the scope of the general practitioner and he will elect to refer the patient to one of the dental specialists.

The *endodontist* treats the nerves of the tooth. The center of a tooth contains one or more canals, depending on the number of roots. Each root has a canal and in it lies the nerve (or pulp) of the tooth. It is not necessary to have the tooth extracted simply because the nerve is involved. The nerve of the tooth can be removed, the canal filled, and the tooth will remain in the mouth as long as the health of the surrounding tissues remains good.

A *periodontist* specializes in treating the surrounding structure of the tooth (periodontium or gums). The periodontist is trained to treat all problems associated with the gums and to bring these tissues back to the state of good health.

The *prosthodontist* is called in if the individual needs fixed bridges, removable partial dentures, or complete dentures, providing the general dentist feels that these services are beyond his scope.

PATIENTS WITH NATURAL TEETH

Patients with natural teeth can expect to keep their teeth throughout their lifetime if they practice good dental hygiene and maintenance. The purpose of the dental profession is to prevent diseases, not repair teeth. The principal areas of concern for those who have natural teeth remaining are periodontal disease (pyorrhea) and tooth decay.

Periodontal disease is one of the oldest-known and one of the most common diseases of man, and affects 75 percent of adults. It is the major cause of tooth loss after thirty-five years of age. However, it is not solely limited to adults; children also have some degree of reversible periodontal disease. In fact, 25 percent of children have destructive periodontal disease with loss of tooth support.

A strong relationship has been shown between dental plaque and periodontal disease. Dental plaque is the furry material you feel on your teeth when you don't brush. It consists mainly of bacteria. Consequently, most clinicians today stress daily meticulous cleaning of teeth with a soft toothbrush and dental floss. If started early enough, the disease process may be reversed and cured. If the disease has progressed so that destruction of supporting gums and bone has occurred, the forms of treatment available may stop the disease process and in some exceptional instances may even result in new support for the tooth.

The best form of treatment, however, is prevention. Today only the patient can prevent periodontal diseases. Someday in the future immunization may be possible or safe plaque-control agents will be discovered.

There are seven warning signs of gum disease:

1. Bleeding gums
2. Bad breath
3. Soft, tender, and swollen gums
4. Evidence of pus at the gum line
5. Loose teeth
6. Shrinking gums
7. Changes in alignment of teeth

If the patient has any of the above symptoms, a dentist should be consulted.

If plaque is not removed daily it will gradually harden into calculus (tartar). This formation helps to force the gums away from the teeth. If the calculus is allowed to form, pockets develop below the gum line, and the disease eventually attacks and destroys the bone that surrounds the teeth. If periodontal disease is allowed to progress, loss of teeth follows.

The best prevention is to remove plaque daily by brushing and flossing. Examine your mouth for the seven warning signs and work with your dentist so you can keep your own teeth for life.

ORAL HYGIENE FOR NATURAL TEETH. There are several ways to clean teeth properly. One is to use a soft toothbrush to thoroughly clean the teeth in the areas of gum tissue close to the teeth. There are many acceptable methods of tooth brushing. Let your dentist show you which one is best for you. Dental floss should be used along with proper brushing. The American Academy of Periodontology recommends the following procedure: Cut off a long piece of floss, and lightly wrap the ends around the middle fingers. Insert the floss between each tooth and, holding it taut, move it gently back and forth past the point where the teeth contact each other. Move the floss with both fingers up and down five or six times on the side of one tooth, going down to the gum line but not into the gum. Repeat on the side of the adjacent tooth. When the floss becomes frayed or soiled, a turn around one middle finger brings up a fresh section. When all the teeth are done, rinse vigorously with water. It is a good idea to rinse your mouth after eating when flossing is not possible.

Other aids, which your dentist may recommend, are designed for use in special instances. Among them are electric toothbrushes, oral irrigating devices, and specially designed brushes.

TOOTH DECAY

Tooth decay afflicts at least 95 percent of all Americans. Bacteria-infested plaque, sugar, and a susceptible tooth are the necessary ingredients for the production of tooth decay. As bacteria in the plaque go to work on the sugar residue in the mouth, they form an acid. This acid is actually held against the tooth by the plaque and will attack the tooth if the tooth is vulnerable.

A person's susceptibility to tooth decay may be largely inherited. Some people seem to have an increased resistance to tooth decay. In other individuals who are highly susceptible to tooth decay more acid is formed in the mouth. But we have no direct method of determining whether a tooth is vulnerable or not.

In theory, to reduce tooth decay we should get rid of or neutralize the acid formed in the mouth. The best way to do this is to lessen the amount of sugar residue because it is a necessary ingredient for acid formation. Acid builds up very quickly in the mouth after eating candy, cookies, and soft drinks. Just rinsing out the mouth with water will cut down on some of the sugar residue that forms in the mouth.

Is there any way the teeth themselves can be toughened against tooth decay? So far, after years of research, only one substance has been discovered that authorities generally agree can toughen the tooth against tooth decay, and that is fluoride.

The best way to reduce tooth decay, then, is to reduce the intake of sweets and remove plaque from your teeth as soon as possible. This can be done by brushing or flossing or a combination of both and by having fluoride applied periodically to your teeth.

PATIENTS WITH COMPLETE DENTURES

In patients who have lost all of their teeth, the remaining structures, primarily the bone that underlies the soft tissues, must be preserved so that the denture has a good foundation upon which to rest. Anyone with complete dentures should rest his mouth for some period each day. The ideal time is probably at night, but if this is not convenient, the patient should remove his dentures for several hours during the day. If the patient wears his dentures continuously, his oral tissues are likely to become inflamed and there is a greater likelihood that the supporting bone will be lost. Patients who wear their dentures at night often grind their teeth. This grinding causes excessive bone loss and tissue irritability. If the bone recedes, the fitting of dentures becomes more difficult.

People with complete dentures should continue to see their dentist at least once a year. During this visit the dentist can evaluate the fit of the dentures and the health of the tissue that the denture rests on, and can spot any potential problems. If the occlusion (bite) of the dentures is incorrect, or if the dentures fit poorly for some other reason, loss of bone may result.

No research studies have been made concerning the "life" of dentures. However, most dentists feel that a denture's life is eight to ten years assuming the dentures were made by a qualified dentist and the patient has had good routine examinations. An important fact to remember is that each succeeding set of dentures is likely to be progressively more difficult for the wearer to adjust to. Bone loss occurs in varying degrees throughout one's life. As the bone decreases, the amount of supporting structure for the denture is reduced. As a result, the fit of the denture is jeopardized. Dentures worn for too long a period of time are similar to old shoes: They may feel very comfortable, but provide no real benefit to the wearer.

A new advancement in dentures is the *overdenture*. This type of denture is a complete denture resting on one or more teeth that have been determined to be in good health. It is necessary to perform root canal therapy (endodontics) on these teeth; after this the teeth are cut off near the gum line. The remaining parts of the teeth act like posts in the ground. They help support the denture, and they help maintain the bone structure. It is possible to place attachments in these teeth that provide mechanical retention for the denture. These teeth, in effect, become natural implants.

Artificial implants as a means of treating patients requiring complete dentures are being explored. On February 24, 1975, *The American Dental Association News* stated that the American Dental Association Council on dental materials and devices reaffirmed its position that dental implants formed from all types of materials were still in need of continued scientific review, and therefore, should not be utilized in routine clinical practice. Until the ADA endorsement comes through, we feel that artificial implants should be regarded as experimental.

Dentures should be cleaned daily. It is important that the dentures be free of calculus (tartar) so that surrounding tissues will not become inflamed. There are ultrasonic cleaners of several types on the market. The wearer places the denture in this device each evening and the denture stains and calculus are removed. An inexpensive solution that works well is a combination of Clorox and Calgon. Place the dentures in a glass of water containing two teaspoons of Calgon and one teaspoon of Clorox. Soak the dentures in this solution for twenty to thirty minutes. We recommend this procedure be done three or four times a week.

There are many products on the market which can be collectively termed *home reliners*. These products are used to temporarily improve stability and retention for ill-fitting dentures. What is important to remember is that these products are intended for use only for short periods of time and then only until a dentist can be consulted to remedy the problem associated with the dentures. Continuous use of these products can lead to increased loss of the supporting bone and to inflammation of the soft tissues that cover the bone. Without care in the use of home reliners, other problems may develop.

ORAL CANCER

The dentist is one of the most reliable sources for detection and diagnosis of oral cancer, which represents approximately 6 percent of all cancer. The earlier oral cancer is detected, the better the chance of a cure. The cure rate of oral cancer lesions is approximately 75 percent. The reason that the percentage of cure is so high is that oral cancer is easier to detect than other forms of cancer. If you notice any unusual type of growth in your mouth, you should see a physician or dentist immediately. Oral lesions can occur in all patients, those with their own teeth, or those with dentures. For this reason, it is especially important for *all* people to have an oral examination at least once a year.

5. Common Eye Problems

Richard Kielar, M.D.

THE three most common eye problems associated with aging are cataracts, glaucoma, and macular degeneration of the retina. Although these problems may occasionally be associated with another disease, most frequently they occur in individuals who otherwise are in good health.

CATARACTS

Within the eye is a lens that is normally crystal clear. As you age, the composition of the lens changes, and the previous clarity becomes clouded. This clouding is termed a *cataract*. It is important to realize that the development of clouding is a normal change occurring during aging. The degree of development of clouding varies with each individual. The degree of clouding also determines how much your vision is blurred. The vast majority of people develop a minor degree of clouding, which has a minimal effect on the clarity of their vision. Mild clouding of the lens may require only a change of glasses to return the clarity of your vision to normal or near normal.

In many instances, the formation of a cataract causes the individual to become nearsighted, so that later in life he seems to have gained "second sight." Many people, as a result, are able to discard their reading glasses.

When progressive clouding of the lens blurs your vision to such a degree that a change of glasses no longer helps, you need to consider the feasibility of a cataract extraction. Whether your vision is decreased to 20/40 or to 20/200 is not important, as visual needs vary with the individual. The most important guideline in making a decision regarding surgery is whether the vision is blurred to such an extent that the individual finds it interfering with his normal life style. When you find that more than minimal restrictions on your activities are required to accommodate your reduced vision you should then seriously consider surgery to remove the cataract.

Modern surgical techniques no longer require that the lens reach an advanced stage of opacification before surgery can be performed. Prolonged hospitalization and immobilization are also no longer necessary.

Although the probability of a successful result is

high in modern-day cataract surgery, unforeseen complications may develop. Thus, before you decide to have a cataract removed you should have a thorough discussion with your eye doctor regarding your visual needs and expectations.

Following cataract surgery your doctor may prescribe spectacle lenses, contact lenses, intraocular lenses, or a combination of these devices. Each has its advantages and disadvantages, and no one method is the best correction for everyone. We still cannot match nature's normal vision perfectly once a cataract has been removed.

GLAUCOMA

Glaucoma is a condition in which the pressure within the eye is elevated, and has resulted in damage to the optic nerve. It usually occurs in both eyes but may occur in one eye several years before the other is involved.

There are many types of glaucoma, but the most common type associated with aging is chronic simple glaucoma, also called open-angle glaucoma. The channels through which fluid flows out of the eye gradually become obstructed, producing a gradual elevation of pressure inside the eyeball. This elevated pressure in time damages the optic nerve which transmits visual impulses to the brain. An initial sign of damage is a decrease in peripheral vision, which is rarely noted by the individual. If not controlled, further constriction of the field of vision may occur—with ultimate blindness.

It is important to realize that this disease produces no symptoms until it is far advanced, and that any damage to the optic nerve is not reversible. Because of this, routine eye examination is the *only* method of early detection of this sneaky disease. Pressure inside the eye is measured with an instrument called a *tonometer*. The procedure is painless, takes only a few seconds, and is part of any routine eye examination. Observation and evaluation of the optic nerve with an instrument called an *ophthalmoscope,* and plotting of your field of vision are other methods employed to evaluate whether elevated pressure has resulted in damage to your eye. It is important to tell your ophthalmologist about *any* medications that you take, as some, particularly corticosteroids (cortisone) and blood pressure medications may worsen the glaucoma.

Open-angle glaucoma is generally treated with a variety of eye drops and pills, and the vast majority of cases can be controlled to prevent further damage to the optic nerve. If medication is prescribed, it is important that your ophthalmologist reviews with you his instructions regarding how to use your medications to make sure they are taken at the appropriate time and administered to the appropriate eye.

Occasionally medication is unsuccessful in controlling intraocular (inside the eye) pressure, in which case an operation will be necessary. The newer surgical techniques are generally successful in controlling intraocular pressure when medication has not been successful.

Open-angle glaucoma is never cured, nor is the damage already done reversible. The goals of treatment are to control intraocular pressure and prevent further damage to the optic nerve. Thus, once the diagnosis of glaucoma is made, periodic checkups by your eye doctor are necessary for your entire life.

MACULAR DEGENERATION OF THE RETINA

The retina is the portion of the eye that is like the film of a camera—it records the visual impulses. It can be divided generally into two areas: (1) the macula, which is a small area we use for fine central vision, and (2) the peripheral retina with which we see no fine details, but which is responsible for side vision which allows us to be aware of our surroundings and move around with ease. Most opthalmologists believe macular degeneration is the result of an inadequate blood supply to the macula. It is not necessarily associated with poor circulation in other parts of the body. Symptoms may vary from a slight blurring or distortion noted in reading, up to difficulty recognizing facial features. Most individuals who have this disease do not have a severe form. Although it generally occurs in both eyes, the severity may vary greatly between the two eyes, and one eye may be affected many years before the other.

No universally accepted medical or surgical treatment exists to prevent progression of the degeneration, but two important facts must be recognized. First of all, the individual *never* goes completely blind. Even in severe cases where central vision is markedly impaired, peripheral vision remains *normal,* and thus your ability to get around is minimally disturbed, if at all. Secondly, there are ways to improve the visual image. These generally consist of magnifying glasses, either for distance or for near vision. Distance magnifiers (telescopes) have limited use as the field of vision is markedly constricted, and the point of focus of the lens is at a fixed distance. Thus as you move around, only objects at a given distance (such as twenty feet) are in focus. Magnifiers for near vision generally consist of spectacles, hand magnifiers, or magnifiers on a stand. Each has advantages and disadvantages. The proper optical correction must be tailored for each person's individual needs. No lens is perfect, and you will need to take a positive outlook and bear with frustration in learning to use these magnifiers to their best advantage. Remember, magnification of print also produces magnification of the distortion and blur produced by this condition.

Several points need to be made that are applicable to all three of these eye problems:

1. All are painless.

2. Prolonged use of your eyes for visual tasks such as reading will have no deleterious effect upon your eyes.

3. There are many more individuals with mild forms of these diseases with minimal visual impairment than those with severe forms of these conditions.

4. Progression, if it does occur, generally is very slow, occurring over a span of many months or years.

Many people will be free of any significant disability from these diseases as they age. For those who have one of these problems, medical science has produced a wide variety of equipment and methods with which to minimize the visual disabilities that may occur, thus continuing useful eyesight for the lifetime of the individual.

6. Problems of Hearing

William W. Green, Ph.D.

ONE of the greatest pleasures for older persons is the enjoyment of being with relatives and friends. The keystone of these relationships is communication. When communication is disturbed by hearing loss, a person's vocational goals, social interactions, and emotional stability can be significantly affected. The isolation brought about by the inability to communicate adequately with friends and relatives can be devastating.

Many individuals seek and receive help in overcoming hearing loss. Unfortunately, many others do not obtain needed assistance, perhaps because they may not know what is available to help them or where services may be obtained. I hope hearing-impaired older persons will use this chapter as a guide to needed assistance.

63

HEARING LOSS

Hearing loss is not an uncommon problem. During 1971 the National Center for Health Statistics conducted a survey that discovered 14.5 million individuals with hearing impairments in the United States. The prevalence of hearing loss relative to other common impairments surveyed by the National Center for Health Statistics that year is striking. When compared to orthopedic impairments (19 million), visual impairments (9.5 million), and other impairments (8 million), over one-fourth of the impairments found were hearing losses. Even more striking are the findings that persons sixty-five and older comprised over 60 percent of those with serious hearing impairments and that the prevalence of hearing loss in nursing homes was five times greater than in the general population. Increased incidence of hearing loss with advancing age is a harsh reality as shown by a 1976 Metropolitan Life Insurance Company report. From age seventeen to sixty-five to seventy-five, the rate of hearing loss increases seventeen times. In the over-seventy-five age group, the rate of loss is 30.6 times greater than for the age seventeen group.

Hearing loss is an insidious problem. Many people ignore or deny the problem in its early stages. Perhaps that is not surprising when one considers that the softest sound that the normal ear can typically detect is 0 decibels of loudness while the loudness of conversational speech is in the 40 to 65 dB range. Thus, a person with a mild hearing loss (*e.g.*, 20 to 30 decibels) will miss soft speech but can get along reasonably well in many conversational settings. Denial of the problem or putting off doing something about it is not uncommon.

Most people do not appreciate the importance of hearing in their everyday lives. Although almost everybody knows that good hearing is essential for learning speech and language and for effective communication, what is less well understood is the importance of hearing as a signaling system and as a mechanism that keeps us in touch with our environment. We are constantly relying on hearing to warn us of approaching danger, *e.g.*, a car horn, a train whistle, a storm. Scant attention is paid to this important protective function of hearing until it is lost. Even less appreciated is the importance of hearing for constant monitoring of the sounds around us. We live in a world that is alive with sounds (television, clock ticking, traffic noise, wind rustling through the trees, children playing, etc.) and we take them for granted. However, when hearing loss eliminates those background sounds we feel isolated and we don't know why. This isolation and the accompanying frustration can be a major problem for the older person.

THE PROCESS OF HEARING

Most of us give little thought to the influence hearing has on our lives until we experience problems with this valuable sense. Moreover, most of us have little understanding of the complex structure of the ear and the intricate process of hearing.

A cross-sectional view of a human ear is presented in Figure 1. In order to understand how the ear functions, it is helpful to consider the ear in three parts: *the outer ear, the middle ear,* and *the inner ear.*

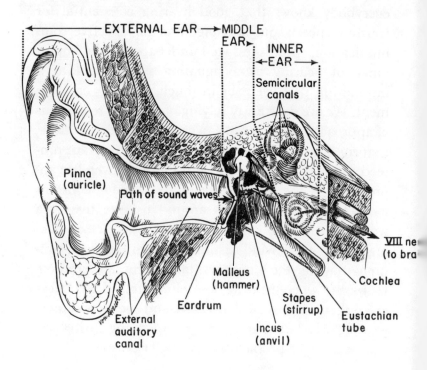

OUTER EAR. The outer ear consists of the pinna, or auricle (the cartilaginous structure on the side of the head), and the external auditory canal. Since the pinna is the only outwardly visible part of the ear, many people think it is the "ear" and overestimate its importance. The function of the pinna is to "collect" sound waves arriving at the ear in a reverse megaphone effect and to focus them into the auditory canal. We actually could hear well without the pinnae providing that we could become accustomed to the cosmetic change.

The auditory canal is approximately one to two inches long in adults and it serves to protect the more vital structures in the ear from traumatic damage or the invasion of foreign objects. There are stiff hairs at the outer edge of the canal that are supposed to prevent foreign objects from entry although it is doubtful that these have much effect. Additionally, the skin lining the outer third of the canal secretes a bitter-tasting wax that functions to trap material and keeps the ear canal and eardrum from drying out. Some individuals are convinced that earwax is "dirt" and they vigorously "dig it out" of the ear. This process is generally unwarranted and can result in irritation and possible infection. The old adage that "you shouldn't put anything smaller than your elbow in your ear" is still good advice. If a problem truly exists with buildup of earwax, consult your physician.

MIDDLE EAR. The structure that serves as a dividing line between the outer and middle ear is the eardrum. This remarkable membrane vibrates when sound waves hit against it. This mechanical vibration is transferred to a chain of three small bones, the malleus (hammer), incus (anvil), and stapes (stirrup). These bones, which are named for their shape and resemblance to objects, carry the vibration across the middle ear cavity to the entrance to the inner ear.

An important structure that is generally considered as part of the middle ear system is the eustachian tube, which extends between the back wall of the throat and the middle ear cavity. This structure opens and closes to regulate the air pressure in the middle ear cavity so that it is equal to the pressure pushing on the outside of the eardrum. We experience how this eustachian tube functions when we descend a hill in a car or dive under water. There is a feeling of pressure or stoppage in the ears which is relieved only when swallowing, yawning, or normal muscle action causes the tube to "pop open."

INNER EAR. The inner ear contains the delicate and intricate structures for balance (semicircular canals), the sense organ for hearing (cochlea), and the peripheral endings of the auditory nerve pathway that leads to the brain (Cranial Nerve VIII). The inner ear is filled with fluid. The semicircular canals do not have any direct influence on hearing. However, because of their close proximity to the cochlea, problems of balance are sometimes associated with hearing loss.

The vibrating stirrup bone moves in and out of an

oval opening to the inner ear and sets up a fluid vibration which travels up and down in the small snail-shell-shaped cochlea. At various places along the way, the vibrating wave stimulates nerve endings of the auditory nerve and an electrical impulse is transmitted to the brain and interpreted.

TYPES OF HEARING LOSS

From the preceding short summary of the structures of the ear and the process of hearing, the complexity of the system becomes obvious. You should therefore not be surprised that hearing loss can occur from any number of conditions or illnesses. There are two basic types of hearing loss that should be considered.

CONDUCTIVE LOSS. Anything that impedes or impairs the functioning of the structures of the outer or middle ear can cause a conductive type of hearing loss. In other words, the mechanical conduction of sound is blocked and the sound must be more intense to overcome the blockage.

The most common cause of conductive hearing loss is middle ear infection. This condition usually begins as a result of a malfunctioning eustachian tube and can sometimes progress to the point where an excessive buildup of middle ear fluid causes perforation of the eardrum. This problem is most common in young children and seldom is the primary cause of hearing loss in the older person.

Another cause of conductive loss is from blockage of the auditory canal by excessive earwax or by a foreign body. If the ear canal is completely blocked, a mild conductive hearing loss can result. However, earwax buildup is often overrated as a reason for hearing loss, particularly by the older person who is bothered by excessive accumulation of wax or the opposite condition of a dry ear canal. There is a tendency to associate the discomfort that is apparent in the ear canal with the hearing loss which is caused by an entirely different condition.

Still another cause of conductive hearing loss is a condition called *otosclerosis*. This results in the formation of a spongy-bony growth around the stapes which progressively impedes its movement and causes gradual deterioration of hearing. Many people with this condition have a stapedectomy, a surgical procedure which often restores hearing to normal.

Conductive hearing losses are usually temporary and the loss will fluctuate in severity depending on the medical condition. Such hearing losses are generally (but not always) medically and/or surgically treatable and with successful treatment, hearing is restored to normal. However, hearing loss in the aged is seldom due to conductive problems.

SENSORI-NEURAL HEARING LOSS. When there is damage or deterioration of the cochlea in the inner ear or of the auditory nerve, the resulting hearing loss is termed *sensori-neural.* This type of problem can occur at any time from illness or disease. The severity of sensori-neural hearing loss is usually greater than in conductive disorders and more extensive rehabilitative treatment is required.

Hearing impairment as a result of advancing age is of the sensori-neural type and is termed *presbycusis.* This is the most common cause of inner ear hearing loss and probably is the most prevalent of all types of hearing loss. It is generally agreed that we experience our best hearing between the ages of eighteen and twenty-six and that gradual deterioration of hearing sensitivity occurs beyond this point. For most of us, the loss becomes noticeable in our sixties, seventies, or eighties. Some few of us will experience less loss than the average and will enjoy good hearing throughout our lifetime.

There appear to be several different aging processes that contribute to presbycusis. Changes in the inner ear bring about deterioration of the nerve cells and structures that are needed to transmit sound from the ear to the brain. Generally, the hearing loss (the inability to hear soft sounds) is greatest for high-pitched sounds. Elderly patients commonly report greater difficulty in hearing higher-pitched women's and children's voices as a result. However, a major result of presbycusis is a reduction in the clarity of what is heard. In addition to his inability to hear soft sounds, the elderly individual often complains that sounds and words are not clear at any loudness. One delightful lady in her seventies explained this problem to me as, "This younger generation doesn't talk as plain as we used to talk." This is often the major complaint of the older patient and, as I will show later, is a major factor in rehabilitation of these patients.

Another major cause of sensori-neural loss is exposure to loud sounds and noise. We are becoming increasingly more concerned about this problem as evidenced by recent government regulations that are designed to control noise in industry (the Occupational Safety and Health Act) and the environmental problems associated with aircraft and other environmental noises. It is well documented that prolonged exposure to noise or brief exposure to a single intense sound may cause damage to the nerve cells in the inner ear. This damage, which generally has a greater effect on hearing high-pitched sounds, may be a large contributor to the hearing loss experienced by older persons, particularly by men who have worked in noisy jobs or who have been exposed to excessive noise in the military service.

Sensori-neural loss can also be caused by a number of other conditions such as childhood illnesses, bacterial infection, viral infection, heredity, drugs, and various disease conditions. These, however, are not the focus of this chapter.

Unlike conductive hearing loss, sensori-neural losses are generally not medically or surgically treatable. In some cases, associated problems such as dizziness can be treated but the sensori-neural loss is not reversible. Another complicating factor is the deterioration of understanding that accompanies most sensori-neural losses. However, there are things that can be done to help those with sensori-neural losses and these will be discussed in detail.

WHO CAN HELP?

The older person with hearing difficulties may not know where help can be found. Moreover, he may be confused about which type of specialist in hearing can offer assistance. There are at least three types of specialists.

THE PHYSICIAN. In many cases, the older person with hearing problems will initially consult with his regular physician. If the problem is medically treatable, this may be the only step necessary in overcoming the problem. In some cases, however, your physician may recommend that you see a physician who specializes in diseases of the ear, nose, and throat—an otolaryngologist. The treatment prescribed may suit the needs of the older person with conductive hearing loss. If the problem is determined to be a sensori-neural loss and therefore not amenable to medical or surgical treatment, the physician should suggest other possibilities for rehabilitation such as a hearing aid, auditory training, and speech-reading and he may refer you to an audiologist or to a hearing aid specialist.

THE AUDIOLOGIST. The audiologist is a hearing specialist specifically trained to evaluate hearing and to provide various types of rehabilitative services. He or she will have at least a master's degree and will hold the Certificate of Clinical Competence from the American Speech and Hearing Association. In some cases, an audiologist works directly with the otolaryngologist and provides thorough testing and auditory rehabilitative services in conjunction with the medical consultation. In other cases, you may be referred to an audiologist in a local hearing and speech clinic to determine whether you need a hearing aid and to provide auditory training and speech-reading services. Many older persons seek the services of an audiologist first and are referred to other specialists as a result of the hearing test findings. The audiologist may provide hearing aids or may refer the older patient to a local hearing aid specialist to fit the recommended aid.

THE HEARING AID SPECIALIST. Hearing aid specialists, or dealers, are those who fit and sell hearing aids. Some of these individuals have formal training related to hearing, others do not. In many states, hearing aid specialists must be licensed to fit and sell hearing aids.

Older persons who have sensori-neural loss may be referred to a hearing aid specialist by a physician or an audiologist with a specific recommendation for a particular hearing aid. The hearing aid specialist will make an earmold, provide the hearing aid, and offer advice on the care of the instrument.

WHAT CAN BE DONE?

We have already alluded to some of the treatments available to the older person with a loss of hearing. It should be apparent that the nature of the loss will dictate the treatment, *i.e.,* conductive losses may respond to medical/surgical treatment; sensori-neural losses require one or more auditory rehabilitative measures.

CONDUCTIVE HEARING LOSS. Someone once philosophized that if you have to have a hearing loss, it is best to have a conductive loss that can be overcome by medical/surgical measures. Unfortunately, such is usually not the case with the older person. In those instances where there is middle ear infection or blockage of the ear canal by wax, this may be successfully treated through medical/surgical measures, but sometimes such treatment only partially satisfies the patient who has a mixed loss—the conductive disability is overcome but the sensori-neural loss remains. The often-heard expression, "If I could only get this wax cleaned out of my ear, I'd be okay," may be a case of hoping for a simple solution to a more complex, permanent sensori-neural problem.

For those older individuals found to have otosclerosis, surgery will largely overcome their problem. However, the percentage of those having this problem is small, and the person may be beyond the optimum age for surgery. On occasion, patients have told me about a neighbor who had surgery for a hearing loss and had hearing restored. They quite obviously hope that a similar solution is available for their problem, but generally this is not the case.

Sometimes hearing aids are recommended for those older individuals who have conductive hearing loss that cannot be overcome through medical/surgical means. This seems to be particularly true for those with advanced otosclerosis that is nonoperable. When hearing aids are used for a conductive hearing loss, the person is often well satisfied since he retains good discrimination ability and the amplification provided by the aid overcomes his loss.

One misconception that repeatedly surfaces is that only those with conductive loss can benefit from a hearing aid. This is based on the assumption that the damaged nerve cells in sensori-neural loss cannot be stimulated by the hearing aid and, therefore, amplification will not suffice. While it is true that those with conductive losses generally do very well with a hearing aid, they usually do not need one because medical/surgical treatments are available to them. On the other hand, many older individuals with sensori-neural loss may use hearing aids with varying degrees of success. In fact, it is estimated that over 95 percent of all hearing aids are sold to those with sensori-neural loss. This misconception about hearing aids is potentially damaging because the older person with a sensori-neural loss is often told that nothing can be done for him. A doctor who makes such a statement usually means only that there is no medical/surgical treatment available. It does not mean that older people with a sensori-neural hearing loss should not try a hearing aid. More times than not, they will be helped by amplification.

SENSORI-NEURAL HEARING LOSS. The sensori-neural hearing loss experienced by older persons interferes with effective communication, so the principal aim of a total rehabilitation program is to improve communication skills. This rehabilitation program may include a hearing aid, auditory training, and speech reading. Additionally, considerable counseling may be required to overcome the emotional/psychological trauma created by the isolation that results from hearing loss. A necessary first step is to have a thorough hearing test to establish the nature of the problem and to fit the rehabilitation program to the person's needs. Then, the choice of rehabilitative procedures becomes clear and individualized.

Hearing Aids: Hearing aids are electronic devices that make sounds louder. A hearing aid is, in a sense, a wearable public address system. In recent years, technological advances have resulted in smaller, more powerful aids with improved quality and fidelity of sound. A hearing aid is not a match for normal hearing but it can in many cases greatly improve communication skills.

However, some individuals with presbycusis are not helped at all by a hearing aid. These individuals usually have poor ability to understand speech and the hearing aid simply makes their misunderstanding louder. In addition, many older persons who report little or no success with hearing aids have expected too much from the aid, that is, they expected it to restore their hearing to normal. Furthermore, some older individuals have bought hearing aids through the mail or gone directly to a hearing aid dealer without any thorough evaluation of their hearing loss. As a result, they purchase the wrong aid, or two aids when one will suffice, or the aid is fitted to the wrong ear. There is no reason for an older person's hearing aid to be "worn in the dresser drawer" if he has been properly evaluated and guided in selecting the hearing aid.

If you have a hearing loss, you undoubtedly have a multitude of questions. Can you benefit from an aid? Should you have two aids? Should you have a body aid, ear level aid, glasses-type or all-in-the-ear model? And so on. The manner in which these and your many other questions are answered and the nature of the specialist providing you with answers are critical issues. Quite frankly, many older persons have been oversold or poorly fitted with hearing aids or misled by false claims and questionable advertising. This has led to recent efforts to control the sale of such devices. The Federal Food and Drug Administration (FDA) has published regulations related to the sale of hearing aids and the Federal Trade Commission (FTC) will publish additional regulations soon. Moreover, licensure boards in various states are attempting to regulate hearing aid sale practices with varying degrees of success.

Speech-reading: When a person experiences hearing loss, he instinctively becomes more attentive to a speaker's lip and facial movements in order to understand what is being said. Most hearing-impaired individuals are unaware that they are "lipreading" or "speech-reading," but it is a natural effort to overcome what is being lost in the hearing process. Speech-reading can be a valuable skill for people with hearing loss as long as it is considered as a supplement and not a complete communication system. Only 30 to 40 percent of the sounds in our language are visible, leaving the speech-reader with many blanks to fill in. And not all people are good speech-readers, even after formal training. Some individuals appear to be more skilled than others in the concentration process necessary for successful speech-reading.

The hearing-impaired older person may benefit

from formal speech-reading training. This training is typically provided by audiologists and speech pathologists through speech and hearing clinics. A person may learn this skill during a series of individual therapy sessions or he might take lessons with a group. These speech-reading lessons should be designed around the experiences and interests of older persons for maximum effectiveness.

Auditory Training: In addition to using a hearing aid and speech-reading, hearing-impaired persons should utilize their remaining hearing to the greatest extent possible. This utilization of residual hearing is the goal of auditory training. Through a series of therapy sessions, the hearing-impaired person is taught to utilize and care for his hearing aid. He also learns how to use environmental cues to assist him in conversational settings. His ability to discriminate sounds and words is sharpened through training. Auditory training can be a valuable part of the total hearing rehabilitation program for older hearing-impaired patients.

BARRIERS TO REHABILITATION

There is little doubt that most older individuals with hearing loss can be helped in many different ways. The degree to which they can be helped is the key issue.

Several factors influence the rehabilitation process.

Some of these factors are directly related to the aging process; others are imposed by society.

A person's age can be a significant factor in hearing rehabilitation. For instance, it can generally be demonstrated that the predominant type of loss among older persons is sensori-neural and therefore not amenable to improvement through medication or surgery. The older person must rely on hearing aids, speech-reading, and auditory training at a time when powers of concentration, attentiveness, visual acuity, and alertness may not be at peak efficiency. The potential for frustration is great and often shows an increase with advancing age.

Another age-related problem that may confront the hearing-impaired individual is the time of onset of the hearing loss. If a person has had the hearing loss from an early age, he has likely adjusted to the loss, to hearing aids, and to their strengths and limitations. However, for the person who sustains the loss in later years, the adjustment may be difficult. For some, the hearing loss interferes with their job performance and this becomes their greatest concern. For the retired individual the social need is predominant.

Motivation is quite often a key factor with hearing-impaired older persons. Many older individuals are not interested in programs for hearing rehabilitation. In many cases, they are brought to the hearing clinic by their spouse or by children who are more motivated than they are, and this often results in a negative attitude and defensiveness. Although this is a difficult starting point, it is critical that a start be made. With better understanding of the hearing problem and proper counseling, the older hearing-impaired individual can often be motivated to function fully in his surroundings and not retreat from them.

One of the more frustrating barriers to hearing rehabilitation of older persons is cost. Many older persons on fixed incomes find it difficult to purchase a hearing aid, and to date the Federal Medicare Program will not pay for hearing aids. Additionally, the costs involved in short- or long-term therapy are often difficult for the older person to bear. Efforts must continue to be made to encourage the federal government, state governments, and health insurers to assist the hearing-impaired older person.

Hearing loss, which is quite prevalent in older persons, can have a significant effect on their quality of life. At a time when communication skills are so greatly needed and appreciated, a hearing loss intervenes. But there are ways to combat hearing loss and there are specialists who can be of assistance. Given the proper encouragement and motivation, the older person can and should enjoy hearing skills sufficient to function in our society.

7. Loss of Memory

James Norton, Ph.D.

THE human memory is one of the marvels of the world. A simple experiment you can do on yourself may convince you how extraordinary it is.

Try to recall some pleasant event from an early period in your life—perhaps something that happened in grammar school, or on a particular Christmas. Now, once you have that in mind, begin to pay attention to the details of the experience. Who was there? Can you visualize them? Perhaps a bit of conversation will come back to you. Can you see the colors of the room, of your clothes? If you are recalling a school event, can you see the teacher, remember her name? Who sat next to you in that school room? Try this little experiment for a minute or so, then continue reading.

What you've been doing, of course, is not unusual. All of us do it from time to time, and some of us are better at it than others. The significance of the experi-

ment is to make us aware of the truly incredible volume of information that we all have lodged in our
brains, simply as a result of being alive. This experiment can be repeated, focusing on different life periods. Again and again we find a wealth of detail, huge
quantities of information to which we usually pay no
attention.

Before the age of widespread literacy, before Mr.
Gutenberg's printing press, this capacity for reminiscence was, in fact, the only source of continuity in culture. The "wise old man" may have been wise mainly
because he was old, but he also provided the only way
to find out about how it was "back then." Now, of
course, we have encyclopedias and television and the
awesome power of human memory impresses us less.
That is too bad, I think, because it is a truly wondrous
thing.

PROBLEMS OF MEMORY

One of the most common observations made by
persons who are aging is that their powers of memory
seem to be declining. This is noted frequently by the
aging person himself, or it may be observed by his
family. For example, on encountering someone whom
you have met already, the person's name will fail to
come to mind. You may return from the grocery store
to find that the sugar, which was the main reason for
going, was not bought. A rather unpleasant letter may

arrive from the electric company, informing you that the bill is delinquent—you forgot to pay it. The telephone might ring and on the other end sit three-fourths of your bridge group; the party had simply slipped your mind.

All of these experiences, or others like them, occur to people of all ages. They are not unique to aging; still, with advancing years, they seem to increase in frequency. The very fact of this increase renders them more than the minor nuisance they were in younger years, and this is a source of some distress. However, you can learn to live with this sort of distress and, in fact, master techniques to improve recall, which I discuss below.

These same difficulties with memory may also engender a more serious sort of distress—the fear that these memory difficulties presage something else, something worse. In the vast majority of cases, the fear is baseless and should be allayed. Not infrequently, an aging patient will ask if he's "losing his mind," or "growing senile." When asked why he thinks this, failing memory is usually the source of concern.

Let me state emphatically that in the vast majority of cases, problems with recall in older persons have no significance other than the fact that they are a personal nuisance. They are not a symptom of something else. They are just what they are—problems with memory, and they are disabling only to the extent that you fail to learn how to cope with them.

In a minority of cases memory problems *are* symptoms of other conditions. These conditions of medical significance fall into three categories: depression, drug intoxication, and diseases of the brain.

Since depression, intoxication, and brain degeneration include memory problems as a symptom, whenever a problem in memory is noted, the doctor should be consulted to rule out these conditions. In the vast majority of cases, however, memory decline is simply a normal problem of aging.

DEPRESSION. Depression is a psychological state that includes feelings of sadness and hopelessness and is associated with difficulty in sleeping, loss of appetite, and loss of weight. Decreased energy is also a part of this state. Depression occurs in people of all ages, but it is frequent in the elderly. It can be either a mental disorder with no external cause, or a reaction to a tragedy or loss. The relatively high frequency of depression in the older person may reflect the fact that loss of loved ones and decreasing activity levels are an inevitable consequence of advancing years. Leaving one's job and associates may be experienced as a loss and elicit depression.

Memory disturbance is one symptom of depression. When a person is significantly depressed, his mind is filled with internal thoughts and worries. As a result, events going on outside are not noticed and not remembered. The person is preoccupied and memory function suffers as a consequence.

Depression is a treatable condition. There are medications that can alleviate it. Electroshock therapy may also be helpful. The important thing for the sufferer is to diagnose the depression and not make the mistake of viewing the memory problem as a normal part of aging. This means that the patient should pay attention to his moods, appetite, and sleep patterns, and be aware that life crises, such as the death of a spouse, may lead to a depressive episode. When memory problems occur in such a context, there is a chance that they are a symptom of depression. If you notice such symptoms in yourself or if you observe them in a loved one, consult your physician.

INTOXICATION. Drug intoxication sounds exotic, associated with jet setters or wild teenagers and not a problem of the aged. This is only partly true. Certainly intentional abuse of narcotics and other drugs is a rarity in aging people, but intoxication can occur inadvertently. Perhaps a patient is taking some medication for blood pressure and has been doing so for years. As he grows older, he finds he has trouble sleeping. Now his daughter also has this trouble and she finds relief using an over-the-counter preparation, so the patient adds this to his routine. The woman next door says she finds a sleeping pill her doctor gives her is very effective, so she passes some of those along. Now sleep is better, but the patient has a hard time waking up. His wife says her diet pills perk her up, so the patient gives those a try. He really has wondered all along, though, if his problems aren't due to inadequate vitamins and minerals, so a heavy dose of some tonic or other is added, along with an occasional decongestant. After a while, the patient's memory grows quite bad and he fears he must be losing his mind. At last, the doctor is consulted.

This fanciful story illustrates what a wide variety of medications can find their way into one person's daily intake. Most of them may have been necessary at one time, but their use may persist long after the reason for which they were prescribed has passed. Furthermore, as people age, their systems become more reactive to drugs, so that the risk of overdose increases with advancing years. (See Chapter 2.) These facts lead to two recommendations for drug use in the aged. First, *do not take medication that has not been prescribed for you.* A drug that is doing your neighbor a world of good may make you quite ill, because of other medication, or because of your own biological makeup. Second, an older patient should routinely see his doctor every six months and go over every drug he is taking. Find out why you are taking each one and see if they are still needed. If you have added a nonprescription drug, let your doctor advise you if it is helpful or potentially harmful. Inadvertent intoxication is a fairly frequent occurrence in older persons and may lead to significant impairment in memory. Careful, periodic review of medications can help you to avoid this problem.

There is another common source of intoxication, alcohol. Tolerance for alcohol declines with advancing years. This means that the older person should decrease the quantity he drinks. If three or four cocktails were consumed daily at age thirty, that should drop to one or two after age sixty. Tolerance for alcohol cannot, of course, be stated in precise, quantitative terms applicable to all people. People differ widely in this regard, but in general as you age, you should be aware that your tolerance will drop and you should adjust your consumption accordingly.

BRAIN DEGENERATION. A third condition that can give rise to memory loss is organic disease of the brain. In these degenerative diseases brain tissue is destroyed, causing not only memory defects, but deterioration in all areas of psychological function. Early diagnosis of these conditions, whose onset is usually insidious, helps both the patient and his family in planning for his care. Regular visits to your doctor are the best way to ensure early discovery. We have no successful treatment for these diseases; fortunately they are rare.

In addition to degenerative diseases, brain tumor and stroke may cause memory defects, but these are usually accompanied by a great many other changes as well. Certainly any abrupt change in psychological function should be brought to the attention of the physician.

STUDIES OF MEMORY

A great deal of research and clinical observation has accumulated over the years in the attempt to discover why some things are remembered and others are not. The problem has been approached from two different but complementary vantage points. On the one hand, researchers have studied the psychology of memory, analyzing the process to see what sorts of stimulus events are important, and what sorts of strategies people use in remembering. On the other hand, researchers have tried to understand what brain activities and regions are critical to memory. There has been progress on both fronts and we hope that, ultimately, the two will come together to give a complete understanding of memory. Let's look at the brain first.

BRAIN AND MEMORY. The first question about the brain and memory concerns what we call *localization.* Is all of the brain involved in memory, or are some regions more important than others? Some of our best information on that question comes to us from a source we'd rather not have—disturbance in memory as a result of disease of the nervous system. Patients with epileptic seizures originating in a region of the brain called the temporal lobe often have a curious symptom as part of their seizures. This symptom is an intense reminiscence of some earlier event. Patients whose seizures originate in other brain regions don't have this symptom. Professor David Clark, chairman of the Department of Neurology at the University of Kentucky, has shared the following case with me which illustrates this point:

This patient was under my care for several years when she was a young married woman. She had developed seizures and in these seizures she always was able to identify the onset because she had exactly the same experience at the onset. That experience was that for a brief instant, she relived an episode that occurred when she was only thirteen years old. She came from a well-to-do family and as a girl she would show horses. The episode she recalled had to do with a fall from a show horse. She was not injured in the fall and there was no reason to believe that the fall had anything to do with her seizures. For a brief instant, she would see above her the horse's belly with the girth of the saddle across it. She could smell the tanbark into which she had fallen. It was a bright summer's day and she could see the sun beaming down. She could hear the calls of the people who were in the grandstand, concerned about her fall. The episode was absolutely complete and total. It represented less than a second of experience, and every time she had one of her seizures, she would have this experience. My colleagues and I were able to demonstrate that this patient had a lesion in her temporal lobe. Fortunately, her seizures were well controlled with medication and she no longer has them.

A second source of information about the brain and memory comes from patients with a disease known as *Korsakoff's Psychosis*. This is a syndrome seen in people with serious and prolonged abuse of alcohol and in persons whose diet, for whatever reason, is extremely deficient in B vitamins. The syndrome includes as its most dramatic feature a profound inability to register new information. Recall for remote events may be perfectly intact, and general intelligence is quite normal, yet these patients recall almost nothing of what happened in the recent past. Professor Raymond Adams of the Harvard Medical School and his associates have studied the brains of a great many such patients at autopsy and they find destruction of brain tissue in the temporal lobe region and in structures related to it.

From these and other sources, then, we can conclude that the temporal lobes and their interconnections are critical factors in the process of memory. As a result, when profound memory loss occurs but there are no signs of other psychological disturbance, dysfunction in the temporal lobes is suspected. Let me emphasize that I am describing here quite abnormal memory function, not common forgetfulness. Similarly, a patient with a temporal lobe seizure does not experience normal reminiscence, but rather a stereotyped, sudden image that is followed by the seizure.

PSYCHOLOGY OF MEMORY. The problem of memory can also be approached from the psychological rather than the neurological side. Many years ago a

German psychologist named Ebbinghaus performed some experiments on himself to try to isolate factors that contributed to memory. Specifically, he memorized lists of trigrams—meaningless bits of pronounceable rubbish like KOT or TUZ. Ebbinghaus wanted to study memory itself, independent of prior experience or education, and felt that meaningless material would be a pure measure. One thing he found was that trigrams at the beginning and end of the list were remembered better than the ones in the middle. This is called an *anchor effect*. Examples in everyday life illustrate this. When listening to a long and dull lecture, or in reading a boring passage you often find you remember how it started and how it ended, while the middle is a blur.

Ebbinghaus found that the lists he studied most recently were recalled better than ones he studied a while ago. This is called the *recency effect* and, again, experience bears it out. You may be able to recall what you did last Tuesday, but not the Tuesday before. This recency principle is complicated, however, and clearly is not a complete explanation. Some memories from long ago can be quite vivid, as I hope our experiment illustrated, while more recent years are much less well recalled. This brings us to a third psychological fact.

Salient events, highlighted ones, are remembered better than nonsalient ones. Related to this is the fact that meaningful material sticks with us better than nonmeaningful. We can remember a seven-word sentence much more easily than a list of seven unrelated words. Ebbinghaus suspected this and that is why he used nonsense words rather than meaningful ones to got a more pure measure of memory. The effect of salience is obvious to all of us. Most people can remember their graduation or wedding day, but would be at a loss to try and recall what happened on that date the year before graduation or marriage.

Two other principles have emerged from psychological study that bear mention. One is that repetition increases memory. Every student knows this, but psychologists have gone to some pains to study this factor in more detail. Finally, things that follow a pattern are remembered better than things that appear at random. Looking one last time at our friend Ebbinghaus' trigrams, lists that are presented in the same order are remembered better than ones that have the same nonsense words, but are presented in varying order.

MEMORY IMPROVEMENT

These facts about memory can be used to help a person whose memory is less effective than it once was. The principles of organization, of anchor effects, saliency, and meaningfulness are all related and imply an important practical device: Things that need to be remembered are more likely to be remembered if they are part of a meaningful totality, of a whole, rather than if they are isolated bits of information. Let us take as an example the problem of remembering a name. Perhaps you are at a party and are introduced to Mr. Smith. The first and primary association in memory is between Mr. Smith's face and his name. When you were twenty-five years old, that single association might have sufficed to lock Mr. Smith's name in memory. At sixty-five years of age, however, this may not be sufficient. (I might note that, at age thirty-five, it is not sufficient for me.) What can you do about that?

Using our principles of saliency and meaningfulness, try to tie Mr. Smith's name to a number of other attributes through conversation. After being introduced to Mr. Smith try to learn something about him by making conversation. It is easier to recall the name if it is associated with a sort of portrait in your mind, rather than being associated only with a face. What does Mr. Smith do? Is he married? Does he have children? Especially, what are his unique attributes? Saliency will help you remember. At a party full of doctors, you are most likely to remember the one advertising executive. That name will stick out while Dr. This and Dr. That recede in a blur. One way to help remember a name, then, is to create a richer impression of the person through conversation, paying special attention to his unique, salient characteristics.

Repetition is also important. After being introduced to Mr. Smith, you might say, "What was your

name again? I missed it." This way, the name will be
repeated. Perhaps, in a few moments, someone else
will approach. Pay attention as Mr. Smith is again introduced, for this is yet a third repetition. It will also
help if you repeat the name to yourself as you look at
Mr. Smith. Later in the evening, when you again encounter Mr. Smith, again repeat his name to yourself,
or make a point to use it when talking to him. Ad-
dressing someone by his name is not only polite, it is
also a helpful memory device.

Patterning and regularity are important in memory. If you go shopping every Monday, you are much
more likely to remember to do it than if you shop just
any day. Days of the week associated with a certain
repeated activity increase the likelihood that the activity will be remembered. This is a simple way to take
advantage of naturally occurring events, the days of
the week, to help you remember. This is also true of
days of the month. You can construct a special kind of
calendar to help remember monthly events, like paying bills. Get a large calendar, big enough to write
things in the spaces for each day. At the beginning of
each month write in the bills to be paid on the proper
day. Better still, put the calendar on a bulletin board
and thumbtack the bill itself to the calendar on the
day it needs to be paid. By checking the calendar each
morning, you will automatically be reminded to pay
the bills and thus avoid an embarrassing note from a
creditor.

Two more general devices will help memory. It is a good idea to make lists of things you have to do, and to check things off as they are accomplished. Everyone is familiar with shopping lists; we use them all the time. As aging occurs, this same general process can be used to remember activities of all sorts. If you carry a list on your trip downtown, you will avoid the exasperating experience of coming back home without making a necessary stop at the drugstore. A second, related device is to carry at all times a small spiral notebook and a pen. Jot down things you need to remember *at the time you think of them.* Don't wait. Waiting is the first step in forgetting. By keeping this little notebook handy, you are always able to remind yourself of what you need to do. If it is something you need to do in the future, write it on your calendar when you get home. Make it a habit to check frequently both your notebook and your calendar. This will keep you on top of things and will help you avoid overlooking appointments, a common problem with many older persons.

In most cases, memory problems are a normal part of aging and are not something about which to be unduly concerned. At sixty-five you cannot run as fast as you did at twenty-five. You find ways to live perfectly well without running, and you can find ways to lessen the problem of a weak memory. Use some of the suggestions I've given, or think up your own devices to aid memory.

One anecdote, also from Dr. Clark, illustrates that problems with recall are common even in aging people who are famous. During his later years the American poet Longfellow was called upon to dedicate a monument to the English poet Wordsworth. In the course of his address, he turned to the assembled crowd and said, "We are gathered here together, my dear friends, to honor the memory of our revered chief, a man who changed the shape of English arts and literature, whose memory we love and revere, but whose name at the moment I do not recall."

It may be a comfort to those aging who find problems with memory, to know that they are in the company of the famous. This lapse of Longfellow's endears him to me because, even in relative youth, I forget names with a frequency that would be alarming, were the problem not so common. Clearly, what we must do is to work at improving our memory, and not squander our mental energies worrying over it.

8. Speech and Language

Joseph P. Fox, Ph.D.

THE one type of behavior that is uniquely human is the ability to communicate verbally. This means that we use a language system that includes a vocabulary and a set of syntactic rules. These syntactic rules govern how different vocabulary words can be arranged with each other to make grammatical sentences.

Humans are capable of language behavior because of the design and complexity of the human brain. Our abilities to learn words, deduce grammatical rules, and to plan specific messages are all related to the activities of the brain, particularly the surface of the brain, or the cerebral cortex.

Our nervous system contains four major systems that support linguistic communication. These four systems underlie the behaviors we commonly call (1) conceptualization, (2) semantics, (3) speech, and (4) the human senses, particularly hearing and vision. Normal human communication requires that these four systems be operating properly; malfunction of one or more of these systems creates significant communication problems. The reverse is also true: All communication problems are related to dysfunctions in one or more of these four systems.

CONCEPTUALIZATION

Conceptualization is a fancy word for *thinking,* but it is important to remember that we learn about our world and think in terms of *concepts.* Concepts are lists of bits of knowledge in our brain that enable us to put objects and actions into categories. When we hear or use words like *chair, glass,* or *run,* we do not generally think of just one chair, glass, or running event. Rather, what we are thinking of is a whole class of objects or events that have some critical features of meaning in common. Needless to say, our conceptual abilities are quite complex, but the fact that we have concepts does not alone make language possible.

You will notice that *language* was not specifically listed as one of the behaviors underlying human communications. The term *language* means the entire linguistic system used by a speaker to communicate, including both the words chosen (semantics) and the speech sounds produced (speech). Therefore, when we discuss semantic and speech-sound production, we are referring to the two divisions of language. In general, language is the tool we use to communicate concepts from our minds to the minds of others.

SEMANTICS

The most complex level of language is that dealing with meaning, or semantics. Having an idea we want to communicate is the first step toward speaking. The second step is choosing the right words to accurately represent that thought in the mind of our listeners. This is the semantic level of language. Two coordinated semantic operations are necessary to create a sentence. First, we must choose the appropriate words (vocabulary) and second, we must put them in the correct arrangement (syntax). Consider the three sentences below:

1. A girl finds a dog.
2. The dog chases the cat.
3. The cat chases the dog.

Sentences 1 and 2 have different meanings because they contain different vocabulary items in the same syntax arrangement. Sentences 2 and 3, however, have different meanings because of different syntactic arrangements of the same vocabulary items. When we listen to sentences from others, our nervous system reverses the process and deduces the vocabulary items and syntactic arrangements from the flow of speech we hear.

When people have difficulty with the semantics of language, they are said to have *aphasia*. They have difficulty saying the right word or putting their words in the correct syntactic order. Contrary to many popular notions, the degree of severity is about the same whether speaking or comprehending.

SPEECH SOUNDS

Thus far we have discussed how normal speakers have ideas (concepts) they want to communicate and begin by pairing their concepts with particular vocabulary items in particular syntactic arrangements. For this message to be transmitted through the air to our listeners the speech sounds for the chosen words must be produced by the tongue, teeth, lips, soft palate, pharynx, and larynx. These structures are the speech "articulators," because their movements in relation to each other create the sounds we call speech.

The process of organizing the sequence of speech sounds and the transmission of these sequences to the muscles is called *motor speech* and is the second component of language. As just suggested, there are two levels of motor speech behavior. The first is the brain's sequencing of motor movements for strings of speech sounds, and the second is the transmission of these commands to the speech articulators. Damage to the first system is called *apraxia of speech* and results in poorly organized speech-sound arrangements. There is no sign of muscle weakness. Damage to the transmission system, however, results in muscle weakness that results in poorly articulated speech (dysarthrias) and possibly impaired voice quality (voice disorders).

Our nervous system also receives speech sounds from others and *automatically* perceives the speech sounds present before our brain decodes the words and syntax. When we are deaf or hard of hearing, the speech of others may be so distorted that our brains simply do not get enough information to understand some or any speech. In some cases, hearing is intact but the mechanisms for perceiving the speech sounds are damaged. In this case the person reacts to sounds in general, but speech sounds are not perceived and therefore sentences are not understood. This problem is called *auditory verbal agnosia.*

MEMORY

The last communication system necessary for normal language that we will discuss is memory. There are generally three types of memory functions required for communication: (1) immediate, (2) short term, and (3) long term.

Immediate memory is required for holding the rapid and multiple sound changes occurring in speech that we perceive as speech sounds. There is evidence that our perceptual system uses information about one speech sound in assisting the decoding of adjacent speech sounds. For example, we still "hear" the sound "t" at the end of the word "bat" even though it may not be articulated.

Short-term memory appears to come into effect with semantic units like words or number sequences. Often the general meaning of sentences is not understood until the last word is "decoded" and related to the rest of the sentence being held in short-term memory. Consider the basic differences in meaning of the following two sentences that are structurally identical, except for the last word.

1. The car was painted by the boy. (The boy did the painting.)
2. The car was painted by the tree. (Someone painted the car next to a tree.)

Short-term memory problems also seem to limit the length of sentences a person can produce. Long-term memory deficits affect communication to the extent that they interfere with conceptualization and message planning or interpretation. Memory losses related to aging are quite variable depending upon the location and severity of damage or malfunctioning, but they involve one or more of the systems just described.

CAUSES OF SPEECH AND LANGUAGE PROBLEMS

It is misleading to imply that the communications problems just discussed are solely of those advancing in age. These same communication problems occur frequently to persons at all ages. Also, most adults retain most of their communicative skills throughout their entire life. It is not, however, misleading to suggest that the changes that occur when one ages do increase the likelihood of developing a significant communication problem.

Many of the communication problems that are more prevalent among the aging are related to some type of damage to or malfunction of the central or peripheral nervous system. These include the brain, the spinal cord, and the peripheral nerves to and from the skeletal muscles and skin. *What* causes the damage or malfunction is often not as important as the area in the nervous system *where* the damage occurs. The destruction of enough tissue to fill one-quarter cubic inch of volume could cause aphasia if it occurs in the posterior left hemisphere, apraxia if in the anterior left hemisphere, problems with spatial orientation if in the right hemisphere, severe dysarthria if in one part of the brain stem, or death if in any number of locations in the brain stem or base of the brain.

Since the cells of the nervous system require large amounts of oxygen, they are most susceptible to damage from lack of oxygen. Oxygen is carried to all parts of the nervous system in the blood, so anything affecting blood supply at any point threatens the continued life of nerve cells supplied by that artery from that point on. If a blockage or cessation of bloodflow occurs in any of the arteries supplying the brain, that is called a *cerebrovascular accident* (CVA), or *stroke* (for more detailed information see Chapter 9). There are a number of bodily changes which occur due to age that tend to increase an older person's chances of having a stroke. First of all, any heart trouble (for example valvular heart disease) could diminish the flow of blood through the brain so that brain function is impaired either temporarily or permanently depending on the degree and length of oxygen deprivation. Enough oxygen may not be getting into the blood or to the cells as a result of pulmonary, metabolic, or infectious disease. Also, blood clots can form in the arteries of the brain, can grow and block the blood flow. These are called "thromboses." Blood clots can form elsewhere in the body (often in the heart), float through the blood stream and finally lodge in an artery in the brain. These kinds of clots are called "embolisms."

As age increases, the inside walls of the arteries throughout the body lose their ability to allow some blood materials to pass through them as easily as usual and a residue builds up. As this material collects, the inside dimensions of the arteries are reduced, thus decreasing the amount of blood that can travel through. This process, called "arteriosclerosis," occurs in virtually all of us, but is more severe in some than others.

As the arteriosclerotic process occurs in arteries of the brain, the chances for a stroke increase. The blood clots can start on the rough edges of this sclerotic plaque and close the artery downstream. If partially blocked arteries are detected before permanent damage has occurred, there are a number of medical or surgical treatments which can significantly reduce the possibility of permanent damage to the nervous system.

Sometimes stroke-like symptoms appear, then disappear after a short period of time (transient ischemic attack). Such symptoms can include any of the speech or language problems already mentioned. If speech or language problems come and go, that is an early warning signal to see a neurologist as soon as possible. In addition to temporary impairments of speech or language behaviors, some other obvious signs of transient ischemic attacks are temporary muscle weakness on one side of the body or the other, changes in touch sensations, loss of balance, impaired orientation, visual problems, memory problems, or problems with intellectual functioning. If these kinds of symptoms occur and do not clear up spontaneously, a completed stroke has occurred and behavioral losses may be permanent.

In addition to cardiopulmonary problems related to aging, other more subtle changes occur. As we age, our brains actually become lighter. This seems to be related to the loss of nerve cells which do not regenerate themselves when damaged or when they die normally due to aging. Only the cells in the peripheral nerves to and from the skeletal muscles grow back when damaged.

The loss of neurons in the brain is also related to

losses in brain functioning. The systems most obviously affected are our sensory awareness and perceptual systems. Both hearing and vision usually undergo considerable reductions in acuity and perceptual skills as age increases. The combined effects of these decreases in sensory transmission systems is a reduction in the recognition of stimuli and in making responses to these stimuli. Thus, reaction times among the aging are slower.

This slower reaction time has a snowballing effect and interferes with a large number of other skills. For example, the elderly score lower on tests of intelligence and memory function, but these scores may actually be due to difficulties in hearing and perceiving spoken directions, or having to study longer visually, rather than to "real" deficits in intellectual or memory functions. It has not been clearly demonstrated which of these alternatives is most accurate.

In general, muscles throughout the body lose some of their mass while aging occurs. Some of this may well be due to nonuse, for those elderly who exercise regularly have no difficulty maintaining strong muscle action. Still there is some structural shrinkage related to aging and even some calcification in cartilage and connective tissues in structures such as the larynx (voice box). This results in changes in voice pitch and quality. Voice quality can also be altered by decreased elasticity of the walls of the pharynx (throat). The greatest alterations of voice are a result of surgery on the larynx to remove malignant cancer cells. Again, it would be misleading to suggest that growing old is the only reason for the higher incidence of oral and laryngeal cancer among the elderly. The overwhelming majority of patients requiring mouth or throat surgery for cancer have a history of smoking and alcohol consumption. The effects on the body from these habits are cumulative, so the final development of cancer simply coincides with being older.

Often the treatment for laryngeal cancer is the complete removal of the larynx (total laryngectomy), leaving the person with no larynx to make a voice for speech. In addition, air no longer passes through the nose and mouth to the lungs. Therefore, the laryngectomee must breathe through a permanent hole (stoma) at the base of the neck. These alterations result in a reduced sense of smell and taste, and require special care of the stoma to prevent respiratory infections or drowning. The laryngectomee can literally drown himself taking a shower, if the stoma is not protected.

The loss of teeth as we age can also have an effect on the clarity of our speech production. Although it is quite possible to have highly intelligible speech with no teeth, some people seem unable to compensate for lost teeth or dental alterations without professional assistance.

There are some oral cancer patients whose tongues must be removed and whose hopes for speech look quite dim. However, working with a speech-language pathologist they can learn ways to compensate with their teeth, lips, and throat to develop unusual sounding, but highly intelligible speech.

TREATMENT FOR SPEECH AND LANGUAGE PROBLEMS

Speech and language behaviors are complex, but we never seem to think about them until they are impaired or lost. Then some of us become so depressed about our inability to continue our lives precisely as before that we want to give up completely. Yet somewhere between perfect sounding speech and language and total despair is a middle ground of functionally effective communication and a different, but rewarding, life. Helping patients with communication problems reach this middle ground is the role of the professional speech-language pathologist.

For the speech-language pathologist's work to be successful he must deal with both the communicatively impaired person and his or her family. Some general principles of treatment apply. First, the speech-language pathologist evaluates the anatomic and physiologic competency of his client and determines which of the normal speech and language skills the client still has or can attain and which will require compensatory behaviors. The actual working and learning is up to the client himself. If fixing a broken verb phrase were as straightforward as fixing a broken arm, the speech-language pathologist would have more direct control over achievement of the desired goals. However, the speech-language pathologist is limited to setting goals and providing guidance and encouragement as the client works his way toward these goals.

If the speech or language problem is related to a stroke, the client must be made aware of several factors. First, after almost every stroke there is some degree of spontaneous recovery where skills not there one day may appear the next. The period of greatest spontaneous recovery is the first month following the onset of the stroke. Additional amounts of spontaneous recovery will occur for the next two months and slightly more perhaps during the next three months. There are no universal rules, and every stroke patient has a unique recovery pattern.

After the first three months following the onset of stroke, however, those disabilities still remaining will probably be permanent disabilities and can be considered the major communicative problems to *overcome*. Therapy is designed to "overcome" problems, not "eliminate" them, because that is basically impossible. The nerve cells in the brain and spinal cord do not replace themselves when they are damaged, so communication systems which include circuits with nonfunctioning nerve cells will continue to malfunction.

The speech-language pathologist prescribes a treatment program that will overcome these disabilities. In this program the client learns to communicate in a *different* way. After strokes resulting in communication problems, most people still try to think and talk in the same way they did before their stroke. However, most patients would improve their poststroke communicative effectiveness if they tried consciously to limit their utterances to two to four words and used words that are easily pictured or demonstrated. Teaching this and similar adjustments in communication strategy and drilling the client in these strategies until he has attained functionally useful communication is the goal of many speech and language treatment programs.

In general, the goal of aphasia therapy is functional understanding and speaking, using words, gestures, writing, or any available skill. The goals for apraxia of speech and dysarthria are for consistently intelligible speech, not necessarily normal-sounding speech. The goal for a laryngectomee would be to learn to develop voicing by injecting air into the esophagus, trapping it, and reversing it to make the esophageal wall vibrate. This is called *esophageal speech,* and is learned by a large number of laryngectomees.

There are ways to compensate for most of the communication disabilities already discussed. Even for persons who are totally speechless because of the severity of their apraxia or dysarthria, there are electronic speech synthesizers commercially available which they can learn to operate manually to produce "computer-type" speech.

Patients who have severe to profound intellectual impairments will not be able to communicate normally. For these people, speech and language serve no useful purpose since they have few concepts they feel any need to communicate. Family members concerned about a severely impaired relative must understand this. The speech-language pathologist should work only with those patients who demonstrate a disparity between what they *want* to communicate and what they *can* communicate. A need to communicate and motivation to satisfy that need have to be present to justify a speech and language treatment program.

WHAT THE FAMILY MUST KNOW. The family of a communicatively impaired person should be aware of several other factors. If a person with normal communicative abilities seems to ignore what we say, or makes related but slightly bizarre responses or seems to struggle with what he wants to say, our internal reactions are that he is rude, crazy, or mentally incompetent. Family members must be on guard not to have these same reactions to their communicatively handicapped relative.

Most people who acquire a communication problem in adulthood feel normal inside and are themselves distressed by how abnormal they may sound or act to others. It is most important that the family learn how to relate directly to the internal normalcy of the handicapped person so that he can feel secure enough to try to improve his outward communicative efforts.

The family can help tremendously by including the communicatively impaired person in the normal activities of the household as much as possible. They can also assist by understanding the nature of the disability as well as what normal skills remain, so their efforts to encourage the patients are not demands for the impossible. Thirdly, they should remain informed about the goals and progress made in speech or language therapy. Linking progress made in the clinic with activities in the home will make these *new* ways of communicating effective and familiar to all concerned.

WHERE TO GET HELP FOR COMMUNICATION PROBLEMS

The treatment programs discussed in this chapter are planned and performed by a professionally certified speech-language pathologist. Most professional speech-language pathologists are members of the American Speech and Hearing Association (ASHA) and have passed the academic training and professional experience requirements for a Certificate of Clinical Competence awarded by ASHA. In addition, many states require professional speech and language pathologists to be licensed.

Certified speech-language pathologists work in a variety of locations. Many universities have training programs in speech-language pathology and audiology and have speech and hearing clinic services available to the public. Many towns and cities have privately operated speech and hearing centers. Other centers are sponsored by parent organizations such as Easter Seals Association or United Cerebral Palsy Association. Many hospitals and medical centers have speech and hearing clinics. Some hospital clinics are open to the public; however, some may be restricted to inpatient treatment. For example, clinics in most training institutions are open to the general public, but VA Medical Center clinics are restricted to those veterans eligible according to patient treatment rules and regulations.

There are increasing numbers of speech-language pathologists going into private practice. Some work as individuals, traveling to the patient, while others have grouped together in adjacent offices and they have clients come to them. Although there are professional speech-language pathologists available for treatment of communicative problems in all areas of the country, more such services are of course available in urban areas.

Those seeking treatment should understand that the speech-language pathologist works with patients who are medically stable or under a physician's medical care. If you or a member of your family experiences a sudden onset of difficulty with speech or language, the first professional to see is a neurologist. Following appropriate medical treatment, if speech or language difficulties persist, the referral to a speech-language pathologist is in order.

Information on speech and language pathology treatment services available throughout the United States can be obtained by writing the Public Information Office, The American Speech and Hearing Association, 10801 Rockville Pike, Rockville, Maryland 20852, or calling them at (202) 897-5700. To save time, you might first call local universities or medical centers and inquire about speech and language services.

One final note should be made about some speech and language problems among the elderly that frequently and needlessly occur. It is the loss of speech and language skills from nonuse. This is based on an important basic principle underlying all of human behavior: *skills which are not used, are lost.* This is just as true for a ten-year-old as it is for a ninety-year-old person. Use your language and keep it in good shape. Be interested in others, learn new words as you hear about them, strive to understand slang terminology, discuss news topics, continue to think actively and your speech and language skills will stay sharp.

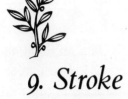

9. *Stroke*

Robert Baumann, M.D.

SHAKESPEARE'S Macbeth comments: "Present fears are less than horrible imaginings." The more we know about a given subject, no matter how fearful that subject, the better able we are to cope with it. So it is with stroke. Armed with knowledge you need not fear that each shake of the hand or slip in memory observed in yourself or others is a manifestation of a previous stroke or a warning of a future stroke.

Stroke is the third most common cause of death in the United States (after heart disease and cancer). Each year 500,000 persons have a stroke and 200,000 persons die as a result. Approximately 80 percent of strokes occur in persons over sixty-five. Fortunately, recent research has increased our understanding of the events leading to a stroke, enabling us to prevent some strokes from occurring and to lessen the disabling effects of some which do occur.

In many older persons changes take place in coordination and mental abilities. Such changes do not necessarily imply a stroke.

A stroke is an injury to a portion of the brain caused by an interruption in the flow of blood to that area. Other terms for stroke in common use are *cerebrovascular accident* (abbreviated CVA), *cerebral thrombosis,* and *cerebral hemorrhage.* Apoplexy is an old-fashioned term seldom used today.

HOW BLOOD REACHES THE BRAIN

Since strokes are related to blood flow, understanding them requires an appreciation of how blood vessels supply the brain. Four large arteries bring blood to the brain. Two of these can be felt on either side of the Adam's apple in the front portion of the neck. Called the carotid arteries, they carry two-thirds of the blood going to the brain. Most of the blood from the carotids goes to the front and top of the brain. The remaining one-third of the blood supply reaches the bottom and back portions of the brain through the vertebral arteries. These arteries are encased in the bony spinal vertebrae and cannot be felt. As they reach the brain, the two vertebral arteries fuse to form one large vessel called the *basilar artery.* The carotid and basilar arteries subdivide into smaller branches which in turn give off additional branches so that every area of the brain receives its portion of blood.

The blood supplies the brain with oxygen and essential nutrients, and removes toxic waste materials such as carbon dioxide.

Since each area of the brain performs specific functions, it is often possible to tell from careful elicitation of the patient's symptoms and a careful examination of the patient's physical disability (signs) which area of the brain is diseased or has been injured. Physicians call this process *localization.* Accurate localization helps the physician arrive at a correct diagnosis. For example, if the back of the brain is injured, a blockage of a carotid artery cannot be the cause of the patient's problem since it is the vertebral arteries that supply the back of the brain.

The determination of which artery is causing a stroke may not always be possible since the arteries supplying the front (carotids) and back (vertebrals) of the brain are interconnected at the base of the brain by the Circle of Willis. In some persons the Circle is anatomically complete and consists of large caliber vessels. Thus, if the blood supply from the basilar artery is diminished, blood from the carotid circulation can traverse the Circle and make up for the lack. In other persons, the Circle is incomplete or has been interrupted because of hardening of the arteries. Then a diminution in basilar flow cannot be made up for by the carotid circulation. When the Circle is incomplete, blockage of a major vessel is considered more likely to result in a stroke. Localization may also be impossible if the damaged area is small or is in a part of the brain whose function is usually "silent."

The brain needs minute-to-minute nourishment. It is always working and cannot store nutrients; even a brief interruption of blood flow can cause damage. Twenty percent of the blood from the heart goes to the brain. *Autoregulation* is the process by which the body ensures that the brain always receives an adequate supply. Even when blood is diverted to the muscles during exercise or to the gut after a large meal, the brain's blood supply is unaffected. In other words, the brain is the last organ to lose its blood supply. For example, after a severe cut, when the body has lost much blood, there will be a diminished flow of blood to the skin (causing pallor) or to muscles, while the blood supply to the brain remains intact. Unfortunately, atherosclerosis and other diseases of arteries can decrease the autoregulatory ability. It is not unusual for some older persons to suffer a stroke after a major injury (such as in an auto accident) or in association with a severe illness (such as pneumonia) in which blood is diverted to other body organs and the autoregulatory process is inadequate to guarantee the brain its necessary flow.

CAUSES OF STROKES

Atherosclerosis, or hardening of the arteries, is the most common cause of stroke and is thought to be a prime factor in at least 60 percent of all strokes. In addition to altering the autoregulatory functions, atherosclerosis produces an accumulation of fatty materials in the walls of arteries. This material is called *atherosclerotic plaque* and can accumulate to the point where it completely fills the hollow inside the artery and stops the flow of blood. It is also a rough area on the otherwise smooth wall of the tube. *Platelets,* which are little blood cells similar to the red and white cells familiar to all, are a part of the mechanism that enables blood to clot; they collect on ragged edges such as those formed by atherosclerotic plaques. Such collections of platelets can speed the rate at which a clot forms and plugs up the artery. A stroke in which a blood clot closes an artery is called a *thrombotic stroke* or a *cerebral thrombosis.*

Even if a clot does not form, such groups of platelets can attain a good size, and their hold on the atherosclerotic plaque can be loosened by the flow of blood. Such a collection of platelets floating free in the bloodstream is called an *embolus.* Since blood flows from arteries of larger diameter to those of smaller diameter, an embolus small enough to float freely in a large vessel can become wedged between the walls of a smaller vessel completely blocking the flow of blood and causing a stroke. In addition to the rough areas caused by atherosclerotic plaques, emboli can also form on rough areas on the inside of the heart after a heart attack, or on rough areas on the edges of the heart valves after attacks of rheumatic fever. Such emboli can also form in chambers of the heart that are not pumping blood efficiently. A stroke in which an embolus closes an artery is called an *embolic stroke*.

A *hemorrhagic stroke* occurs when a blood vessel in the brain breaks and allows blood to enter and damage brain tissue. Such a break usually occurs at a weak point in the wall of the blood vessel; these weak areas can be present from birth. Other weak areas develop because the wall of the vessel has been injured. This frequently occurs as the result of high blood pressure, and is one of the consequences of allowing elevated blood pressure to persist over a number of years.

WHAT HAPPENS DURING AND AFTER A STROKE

All types of strokes have certain features in common. First, strokes tend to happen suddenly. Many occur instantaneously, while others take place in minutes or hours. It is unusual for a stroke to continue to worsen over more than twenty-four hours. Second, most stroke patients who survive their stroke remain unchanged for a period of time immediately after the stroke (plateau) and then improve. The period of plateau may be hours or days. Improvement can occur slowly or rapidly and can continue for as long as six months to a year. The degree of improvement varies from person to person and may be so slight as to be almost imperceptible or so great as to remove all signs that a stroke had taken place.

A stroke usually causes major alterations in abilities. It can cause blindness in one eye, or the inability to see to one side. It can cause weakness of an arm and/or a leg (usually on the same side of the body) or of the face. It can interfere with speech, memory, and other intellectual functions. The severity of the disability and the degree of improvement depend on how many brain cells have been injured, how severely they have been injured, and whether other brain cells can take over their functions. Because of the period of improvement that occurs after most strokes, it is often impossible for the physician to predict how well the patient will fare. An accurate description of the patient's ultimate ability to walk, talk, resume household activities, or return to work may not be possible for four to six months after the onset of the stroke.

While all types of strokes have some features in common, there are also some differences. Embolic and thrombotic strokes are seldom associated with pain though some patients may have a mild headache. On the other hand, hemorrhagic strokes can be associated with severe headache and inability to bend the head forward so that the chin cannot touch the chest (stiff neck). Thrombotic strokes often occur at night. The person feels perfectly well at bedtime and awakens with a paralyzed arm and leg (or other disability). In contrast, both embolic and hemorrhagic strokes tend to strike while people are up and active, perhaps occurring while mowing the lawn or playing golf.

A *transient ischemic attack* is a special type of thrombotic or embolic stroke, the effects of which last only a brief period. By definition the symptoms cannot last longer than twenty-four hours. Most actually last only minutes or at most a few hours. The word *ischemic* refers to a deficiency in blood flow. Other than its brief duration, it has the same characteristics as other thrombotic or embolic strokes. Transient ischemic attacks are of special interest because between one-fourth and one-third of the time they are harbingers of a future stroke that will produce a more lasting disability. It is important that your physician be aware of any symptoms of transient ischemic attacks. Vision may be poor in one eye, and at the same time you may feel a weakness or numbness in the limbs opposite the blurred eye, or a portion of your face might become weak or numb. Researchers are looking for ways to treat persons with transient ischemic attacks to prevent a more severe stroke from occurring. For many years blood thinners (anticoagulants) have been used; more recently drugs that prevent platelets from clumping together on rough surfaces are being tried. It appears that many of these drugs can prevent the occurrence of further transient ischemic attacks. Whether they can prevent a more serious stroke remains to be seen.

It has recently been recognized that transient ischemic attacks and some other strokes are associated with a narrowing (stenosis) of the portion of the carotid artery which is in the neck. This narrowing is usually due to an atherosclerotic plaque. It is possible to remove this stenosis by a surgical procedure called *carotid endarterectomy,* and many of the patients who have had this operation have not had any further transient ischemic attacks. It is hoped that patients who have had such surgery will also be protected against further, more severe strokes.

PREVENTING A STROKE

Many strokes can be prevented. Untreated high blood pressure is the most important and most common cause of stroke. In one study 85 percent of all persons who had a stroke had abnormal blood pressure. The chance of having a stroke is directly related to the height of the blood pressure—the higher the blood pressure, the greater the risk of having a stroke. Obtaining treatment and lowering blood pressure decrease the risk of having a stroke. Even someone who has been hypertensive for many years or who has hypertension and has already had one stroke, can potentially benefit from antihypertensive therapy which lowers blood pressure.

The occurrence of stroke is also related to the presence of atherosclerosis. Changes in habits and life style leading to less atherosclerosis should help prevent strokes. Avoiding cigarettes, exercising regularly, and eating a prudent diet should all be of value. Obtaining appropriate treatment for diseases, such as diabetes mellitus, which are associated with an increased rate of atherosclerosis, should also help. Unfortunately, atherosclerosis is a slowly progressive disorder that cannot be rapidly reversed. Therefore, these measures are unlikely to help persons who have already had a stroke or who are far advanced in years.

Finally the appropriate treatment of conditions that can lead to embolic strokes should help decrease the occurrence of strokes. These conditions include heart attacks, damage to heart valves (especially from rheumatic fever), and irregularities in heart rhythm that promote the formation of clots, especially in the left heart chambers which supply blood directly to the brain.

TREATMENT DURING AND AFTER A STROKE

There are some practical measures that can be taken when a person has a stroke, and it is good to be aware of them. When a person has a stroke, those with him should insure that he gets prompt medical attention. In the meantime, it is important to protect him from further injury to himself because of the loss of function. For example, if a leg is weak or his gait unsteady, he should sit down to avoid taking a fall. If he has trouble swallowing and saliva is accumulating in his mouth, he should be laid down on his side with his face down so the saliva can drain from his mouth. Be aware that a person who has had a stroke may be unable to talk or to pronounce words correctly. All of this is frightening; you can help by remaining calm and speaking reassuringly. Persons who have suffered a stroke may have trouble understanding what is said to them. Speak slowly and use gestures. Vague generalizations such as, "Don't worry; everything will be all right," are less reassuring than more realistic statements of fact coupled with a plan of action: "We understand that you don't feel well. We are calling the doctor and will then take you to the hospital."

Those who were with the patient can be especially helpful when talking with the doctor. There are a number of things a physician can do for a person who appears to have just had a stroke, but he needs to know exactly what happened to the patient. A careful physical examination and appropriate tests will help to determine whether the person's disability is caused by a stroke or by infection, brain tumor, or some other disorder. Elevated blood pressure, irregularities of heart rhythm, or other associated illnesses require appropriate treatment. In some circumstances an anticoagulant may be prescribed to prevent the stroke from becoming worse.

THERAPY AFTER A STROKE

Most physicians ask their stroke patients to resume activities such as sitting and walking as soon after the stroke as possible. The major limiting factor is the patient's degree of disability. A patient with a paralyzed or numb leg may be unable to walk until further re-covery occurs. Similarly, speech therapy and physical therapy can often be started a day or two after the stroke. Physical therapy can help keep an arm or leg limber until strength returns and normal usage is again possible. The physical therapist can also teach patients with residual weakness or lack of coordination how to use their remaining abilities effectively. The therapist will acquaint the patient with a variety of aids, from wheelchairs and walkers to specially de-signed eating utensils and zipper pulls. The ultimate goal is maximum independence.

Loss of the ability to communicate freely is partic-ularly upsetting to the stroke victim. The speech therapist plays an important role in helping the pa-tient and the patient's family cope with this disability. Speech therapy helps the patient express himself more clearly. In addition, the speech therapist is able to suggest ways in which family and friends can better communicate with persons unable to fully understand what is said to them.

DISABILITIES NOT CAUSED BY A STROKE

Since strokes are so common, it has been popular to explain many disabilities occurring in late middle age or later as being the result of small strokes or hard-ening of the arteries. In general, such a diagnosis is in-correct and has caused many persons unnecessary worry. A tremor of the hands appears in many persons as they grow older. When associated with head nodding and when it occurs in a person who retains a normal ability to move about, it is often hereditary. This disorder is called *essential tremor* and bears no relation to stroke. It can be socially embarrassing, but seldom causes much disability. Many persons with this disorder obtain relief from a new drug, propranolol. Other persons with tremor who also have stiffness with a slowing of their movements and a decrease in their facial expression may have Parkinson's disease (shaking palsy). Several new drugs, including L-dopa, are effective in treating this disorder.

As they get older, many persons find it more difficult to learn new information and have some difficulty remembering names, events, and the like. This seldom has any clear relationship to atherosclerosis except that it occurs in those whose age makes atherosclerosis common. It is neither a warning sign of imminent stroke nor a reliable indication that a "silent" stroke has taken place. This problem is sometimes related to medication—the person is taking too much or too many different medicines—or to the presence of a significant untreated illness. Whatever the reason, a visit to the doctor is indicated.

Sometimes the loss of memory progresses rapidly over a period of months and the person becomes senile. This also is seldom related to stroke or atherosclerosis. Some of these patients may have a benign brain tumor or a blood clot on the brain and can respond to appropriate treatment. Many such patients have Alzheimer's disease, the cause of which is currently unknown. While no treatment is available, the disease is the subject of considerable new research.

Stroke is a complex disorder with several different causes. Recent research suggests that the effective treatment of high blood pressure and better prevention of atherosclerosis will prevent many strokes from occurring. Current research is seeking more effective forms of treatment for those persons who suffer a stroke. As medical research becomes more and more sophisticated, it seems certain that better means of preventing strokes and of treating them will be found.

10. Low Back Pain

Thomas Brower, M.D.

A WOMAN has been defined as "a chronically con-
stipated biped with low back pain." Such a statement
will no doubt bring a smirk from the male and arouse
the ire of every female.

Low back pain is not, in fact, limited to women.
Indeed 65 percent of all members of modern society
will suffer from it sometime during their lifetime. To
my parents, *lumbago* was an accepted and sympatheti-
cally understood term for this condition. It seemed as
ubiquitous as the common cold: a transient ailment
that symbolized the frailty of mankind. But for the
normally active, painfree, middle-aged individual who
is "laid low" by unexplainable, immobilizing low
back pain, the experience can be maddening and
frightening.

DEFINITION AND ANATOMY

The area of the anatomy commonly called the *low back,* or *small of the back,* is that region of the spine between the ribs and the pelvis shown in Figure 2.

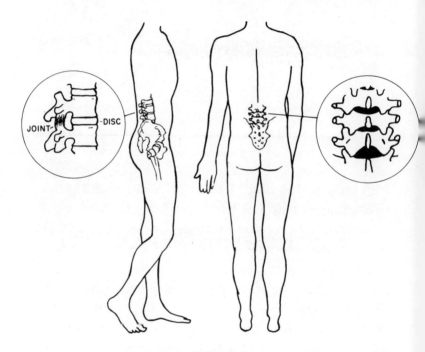

FIGURE 2

The low back. The enlargements show side and back views of a few vertebrae.

Almost all of the pain in this area is caused by the many joints in the lumbar spine, that portion of the spinal column from the chest to the pelvis. Between each vertebral body there is a cushion of fibrous tissue and cartilage (gristle) called the *disc*. Maturity commonly brings deterioration and narrowing of this cushion or joint. If this joint or disc undergoes change, the joints in the back of the spinal column are abnormally stressed, for they are all interrelated to allow bending and twisting of the trunk. To complicate

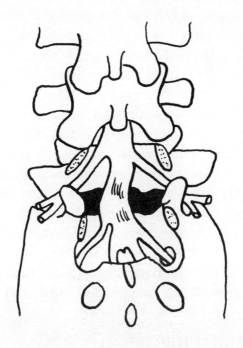

FIGURE 3

The lower lumbar vertebrae as viewed from the back. The black area represents the disc. Should the disc push backward or to the sides the adjacent nerves can become compressed.

matters, the large nerves that go down to the legs and feet run close to these joints (Fig. 3). Should any of these joints become inflamed, the adjacent nerves can become compressed or irritated, resulting in pain almost anywhere from the low back to the foot.

Finally, running up and down the back and sides of the lumbar spine are many heavy muscles providing both stability and control of the backbone or spine. These muscles extend across the flank from the rib cage to the pelvis. Few people appreciate the great importance of the abdominal muscles on the stability of the lower spine. These muscles give control to the front of the spine to balance the muscles we can feel behind the spine. Weakness of the abdominal or belly muscles alters the mechanics of the spine and even the way we walk. Witness the backward tilt of the pregnant woman and her waddling gait. A similar situation, unfortunately less transitory, occurs in the obese male whose protruding abdomen imitates full-term pregnancy. Both the pregnant female and the obese male must lean backward to stay upright. The resultant arching of the low back causes pain. Restoration of normal musculature and posture usually relieves it.

WHERE IT HURTS

Low back pain frequently appears as nothing more or less than pain in the lower part of the back—the small of the back. But with equal frequency people

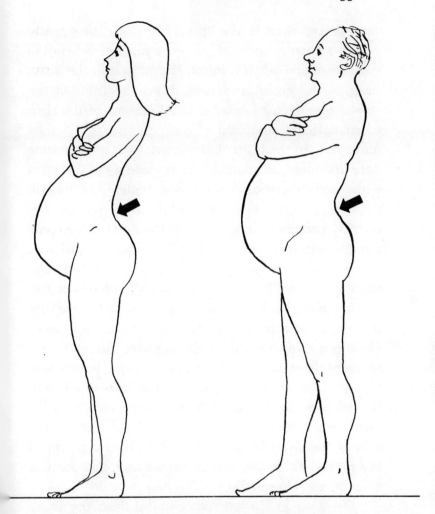

FIGURE 4

A pregnant female and an obese male. To stand erect the individual must lean backward to counterbalance the forward-placed weight. This results in back pain.

complain of pain in the "hip," although the average person has no concept of *where* the hip is or where the pain originates when it hurts. Hip pain is in the front, deep in the groin, and runs down the front of the thigh. The doctor knows that 99 percent of the time when patients complain of pain in the "hip," they mean pain in the buttock. I can understand that some patients might be reluctant to initiate a conversation with their physician with the statement, "I have a pain in the ass," but that's where back pain is frequently perceived. The source is the nerves that come out of the lower spine and supply the pain sensation to the muscles and skin of the buttock. Unfortunately, the location of this pain and its frequent relation to motion of the back and pelvis led many to believe that it was due to abnormal motion in the sacroiliac joint. (This is a joint formed by the sacrum, the lowest extreme of the spine, and the pelvis.) Indeed, for decades doctors manipulated, injected, surgically fused, and braced this joint in an effort to relieve such pain. In fact, the sacroiliac joint is so strong that it can be rent only if one is hit by a truck or falls from a height of several stories. So you can forget the sacroiliac joint as a significant cause of buttock pain.

The pain in the buttock coming from the lower spine is called *referred* pain. Referred pain from the low back goes not only to the buttock but also down the back of the thigh to the knee. It may go around the buttock or flank into the groin. Characteristically, mechanical (caused by movement) low back pain is made worse by activity, diminished by reclining.

THE CASE OF ACUTE LOW BACK PAIN

A middle-aged male bends over to pick up a pencil from the floor, screams in pain, falls to his knees, then lies on the floor begging for help. He states he has severe pain and "spasms" in his low back and cannot move. After three days of severe pain and "spasms" while lying flat (in bed or on the floor) he perceives only a deep ache in the lower back, and he is now able to move carefully and get out of bed. He walks "gingerly," guarding pelvic and back motion. After seven to ten days the ache goes away and he returns to his normal activities.

An episode of this type is referred to as *acute low back pain,* or *lumbago.* Some doctors may offer the sufferer an erudite-sounding diagnosis such as *acute lumbosacral sprain, acute facet syndrome, acute fibromyositis,* or *instability of the lumbosacral joint.* I must confess, however, that I do not know the cause of this man's complaint, and I doubt that anybody knows the cause since this type of back pain does not result in death and so we cannot obtain autopsy material to study it.

It might be helpful to identify what we know does *not* cause acute mechanical back pain. It isn't a muscle pull; it isn't a sacroiliac dislocation; it is not a completely ruptured disc, nor prostatitis, a fallen kidney, or a tilted uterus. All of these have been accused and found innocent.

Logic would lead us to assume that this man caused a joint alteration in the lower spine that was self-limited by a few days of bed rest. The muscle spasm is Mother Nature's way of preventing the joint from moving. The individual accomplishes the same thing by lying still for a few days.

CHRONIC LOW BACK PAIN

Chronic low back pain seems to be the most common affliction of advanced societies. Indeed, in many states 80 percent of Workmen's Compensation funds are spent on people who can't work because of low back pain.

One of the signs of maturity is the realization that prolonged or repeated bending and lifting result in stiffness and pain in the low back or buttock. At the age of forty-five I laid a basement tile floor. After three to four hours on my hands and knees I finished the job and then realized I couldn't stand upright. As I backed up to a wall to regain the erect position, I realized my youth had fled. I was mature.

Chronic low back pain tends to creep up on us. Many people manage to live with it fairly well once they have learned to avoid certain situations like standing for a long time while shopping or at a cocktail party, or anything that requires bending and lifting. Rest in the reclined position helps relieve the pain. At other times, physical activity may relieve the pain but cause stiffness and pain later.

The cause of chronic low back pain seems to be degenerative changes in the discs of the spine and/or alterations of the smaller joints in the back of the vertebrae. These degenerative changes seem to begin by the third decade of life. The complaint of low back pain is most common after age thirty, statistically reaching a peak in the forties and then subsiding. Peculiarly enough, the changes seen on X-ray films that indicate degenerative arthritis increase with age in strictly linear fashion—the older the patient, the more changes seen on X-ray film. But the extent of changes seen on X rays do not necessarily correlate to the person's perception of pain.

In addition to the degenerative changes of life as a cause of low back pain, the emotional stresses of life make a great contribution to this disease. Patients disgustedly state, "The doctor says it's all in my head." This is probably a misrepresentation of the physician's statement, but after years of seeing thousands of patients with back pain one must be impressed by the emotional aspect of the condition. It is rather common for the doctor to hear the patient complain, "I have had back pain day and night for two years and I haven't slept a wink for six months." It is extremely rare for any pain to last constantly for two years and the lack of sleep certainly must be slightly exaggerated. Indeed, back pain is frequently accompanied by depression. The puzzle is whether the mental depression caused the back pain or vice versa.

THE DOCTOR'S EXAMINATION

When the physician sees a patient with low back pain, he will first take a history from the patient. Even with the sophisticated testing devices now available, an accurate history still leads to the diagnosis 90 percent of the time. The greatest wisdom I ever received in medical school was the statement, "Listen to a patient long enough and he'll tell you what is wrong with him. Listen ten minutes longer and he'll tell you what to do about it."

When you see your doctor for your back pain, here are the questions he is likely to ask you:

How long have you had the pain?
(From this he learns whether the problem is acute or chronic)

Where is the pain?
(Low back, buttock, thigh, etc.)

How did the pain start?
(Gradual onset or acute)

Was it related to activity?
(Did the pain follow lifting, bending, a fall, etc.?)

Is the pain increased by activity?
(Lifting, bending, twisting—thus mechanical in nature)

Is the pain relieved by lying down?
(Again indicating a mechanical pain)

The doctor, of course, will enlarge upon or vary the above questions, but within a few moments he will have an opinion as to whether the pain is of mechanical origin (therefore due to degenerative change, some congenital malformation, arthritis, etc.) or whether it is nonmechanical (infection, tumor, etc.).

Next, the doctor will ask about your medical history and about problems with the various systems of the body (ear, nose, throat, chest, heart, stomach, urinary systems, etc.).

Upon completion of the history the doctor will do a physical examination. Besides the usual observations he will check the motion of the spine, chest expansion, look for symmetry of the trunk, feel for tender areas, check the motion of the major joints, and check the tendon reflexes of the extremities and muscle strength.

Upon completion of the history and physical examination the doctor may order an X-ray examination of the lower back (lumbar spine).

Your visit to the doctor has been time-consuming and expensive. It also is disconcerting to learn that, in the majority of cases, no specific cause of the back pain will be identified. When I confess this to some patients, they become irate and exclaim, "What? I spent all that time and money and you didn't find anything wrong with me?"

The doctor and patient do *learn* something. The

patient is obviously concerned that the back pain may be the harbinger of cancer, debilitating arthritis, or some unknown malady that will shorten life or lead to confinement in a wheelchair. These are all real concerns. The doctor can reassure the patient that he or she has none of these problems. That alone should be worth the time and investment.

SELF-HELP FOR BACK PAIN

ACUTE BACK PAIN. The sudden onset of incapacitating low back pain is frightening to the inexperienced. The patient is almost always confined to the reclined position in bed, on the couch, or on the floor. As long as the bladder works normally, the muscles of the legs work so that the toes, ankles, knees, and hips can be moved (albeit accentuating the pain), and the skin of the legs and feet feel normal, no great tragedy has occurred. Three days of rest in whatever position is most comfortable should relieve the severe pain. After three days the individual usually finds that he or she can walk, although cautiously.

CHRONIC LOW BACK PAIN. The nagging backache can be made tolerable by the following:

1. Do lose weight if overweight.
2. Do squat or lift by keeping the back straight and bending the knees.

3. Do exercises when the pain allows. These exercises, shown in Figures 5, 6, and 7, are aimed at strengthening the abdominal muscles and flattening the "sway" in the lower back.

4. Do not bend forward from the hips when lifting anything.

5. Do not do exercises requiring bending to touch the floor from a standing position.

6. Do not ride in or drive a car for long hours. If riding in a car is necessary, stop every hour or so and move about.

Using these few simple guidelines, perhaps you can reduce the discomfort caused by those "nagging back aches."

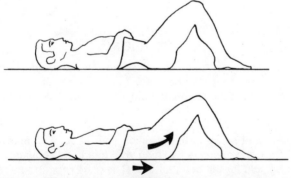

FIGURE 5

This exercise is the "pelvic tilt." Its purpose is to flatten the curve in the lower back. It requires tightening of the buttock and abdominal muscles to force the lower back against the floor. Lie on your back. Tense buttocks and abdominal muscles forcing lower back against the floor. Hold for 5 seconds. Relax.

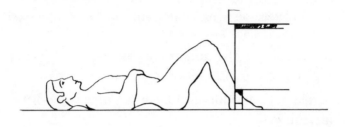

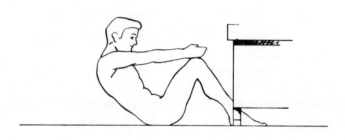

FIGURE 6

This exercise is a "bent knee" sit-up. The hips and knees are flexed and the feet may be placed under a couch. The hips are flexed to reduce the action of a big muscle passing from the pelvis to the thigh. The aim of the exercise is to strengthen the abdominal muscles.

If you can't sit up in this position your abdominal muscles are weak. Start the exercise by lifting your head and shoulders off the floor and hold for the count of five. Relax and repeat. After several sessions of six to ten repetitions you will develop the strength to do a sit-up. Keep working until you can do ten to twenty sit-ups. This exercise can now be enhanced by touching the right elbow to the left knee and vice versa. This variation strengthens the muscles that pass obliquely across the abdomen.

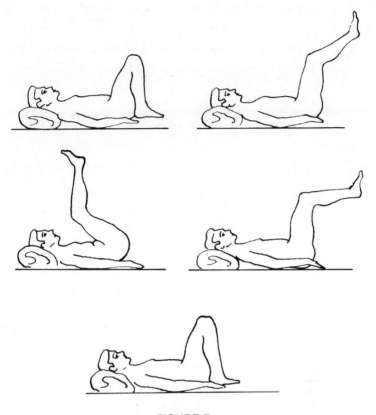

FIGURE 7

Lie on the floor or bed with knees and thighs flexed. Straighten the knees and further flex the thighs. Repeat ten to twenty times. Do this three to four times daily. A variation of this exercise is to flex the thighs and grasp the knees with the clutched forearms and press the thighs on the abdomen. The latter is "self-manipulation" of the lower spine.

Do not lift legs with knees straightened. This accentuates back pain.

However, if your back pain is constant, related to activity, and does not improve with a few days' rest, or if your back pain is accompanied by or precedes pain down the leg to the foot, you should seek medical help.

11. Physical Exercise

Pentti Teraslinna, Ph.D.

THERE is no scientific evidence yet that the theoretical life span of the human species can be increased, but there is ample evidence that the later years can be made more independent, enjoyable, and even productive. This evidence has been gathered in investigations into one of the major characteristics of the aging process, namely the biologically related changes in life functions.

We base our daily living habits on how our body functions. To be able to move effortlessly is basic to a happy life at any age, but its importance becomes most evident with advancing age. We have found that physiological functions in the elderly decrease in direct proportion to a decrease in daily physical activity.

Although exercise will not abolish old age, it may

make it happen later. These extra years of physical activity mean joy of living, not dependence. Unless you have completely lost your health and spirit, it is never too late to start.

The idea of engaging in physical activity or exercise after middle age is rather new, although some of us have heard about "old folks'" exercise clubs in some European countries. We have also heard about the exceptional people who participate in running marathons and other sports until their eighties and nineties. But the value of physical exercise for the average nonathlete is only now becoming widely acknowledged.

Several scientific studies have probed the relation of exercise to health and longevity. Information coming in from various fields, ranging from epidemiology to cellular function, seems to confirm that physical exercise after middle age has definite value.

However, it is impossible to give universally applicable advice about personal exercise programs because of the uniqueness of our backgrounds, both genetic and environmental. With advancing age, we become even more heterogeneous and diverse. Physical activity programs must be individually designed to fit the person's need, and this is not possible without personal consultation. Therefore, in this chapter I provide only basic, general information about the benefits of exercise, rather than detailed instructions on how to exercise.

WHAT IS EXERCISE?

We think first of the traditional competitive school sports. Whatever the athletes do is exercise; it's something that we like to watch perhaps but not participate in. If we think of exercise as a competition, we want to avoid it because we assume we have no chance of winning. Or we may remember how bored we were in our mandatory high school or college physical education class.

By defining exercise in its basic forms, however, we view it as something other than a physical activity needed to build up the skill to compete successfully in sports. Exercise on a noncompetitive basis is something we are all capable of participating in, in some form or other.

There are three basic components to exercise: flexibility, strength, and endurance. Of these three, the most valuable to maintaining health is endurance because this activity develops cardiopulmonary and cardiovascular fitness. The endurance exercises cannot be performed without the involvement of increased heart, lung, and blood vessel function, and that involvement gives the exercise its superior value in enhancing health.

It is necessary to mention briefly the contribution of flexibility and strength to exercise. The more flexible our joints remain, the larger the range of motion around the joints, the better able we are to move and perform daily activities. We can increase flexibility by stretching our joints throughout their range of motion.

Strength, on the other hand, refers to muscle tension developed in a single muscle or muscle group to perform a task. The larger the muscle, the more tension it usually can develop. There are two types of strength activities. One is a sudden movement that requires only a second or less time, getting up from a chair or lifting a grocery bag from a cart to the car trunk. Sustained muscle tension, carrying the bag a longer distance from the store to the home, is the second type of strength activity. The difference in these strengths is the *time* that the muscles maintain tension without relaxing. Obviously, a certain amount of strength is necessary for independent everyday living; when strength training is needed, it should involve the first type, short rhythmic contractions rather than sustained. Sustained contractions will block blood circulation and may raise blood pressure.

ENDURANCE EXERCISES

Understanding exactly how endurance exercises work to build and maintain good health requires an understanding of the complexities of human physiology. Obviously, I am not going to attempt anything of the kind. But it is important that you understand one area of physiology: *basal metabolism.* Basal metabolism refers to the amount of energy that is needed for our body to stay alive. It consists mostly of biochemical re-actions that produce heat as well as a small amount of kinetic energy required for resting heart function, lung ventilation, and smooth muscle work. All this activity is autoregulated; *i.e.*, it happens without any conscious effort. We do not need to use willpower to intitiate or maintain the bodily activities needed to stay alive. Most healthy people are totally unaware of basal metabolic activities.

However, if we have the willpower to increase our muscle metabolism and maintain it for some length of time, that is, to engage in the endurance type of physical activity, we become aware of how the main muscle metabolism support-systems function. We learn that in order to maintain increased muscle metabolism, the muscles need oxygen and certain chemicals. We notice that our heart beats more rapidly and our breathing becomes deeper, in answer to demands by the body. Our body becomes warmer, and sweats to eliminate the excess heat produced by muscle metabolism. These are simple signs of the highly sophisticated way our vital organs function to sustain a higher level of muscle metabolism. Practically the whole body is af-fected to a certain degree.

When we initiate and sustain such a higher level of activity, we consciously learn to tolerate the accom-panying feeling of strain. In addition, in proportion to the intensity of the exercise, the activity of the auto-nomic nervous system (that part of the nervous system that governs involuntary actions) increases, as does that of the many endocrine glands. Lungs, heart, blood, and blood vessels act together to speed the transportation of more oxygen and fuel to the muscles. Even fat is mobilized, and the liver, which regulates fuel supply and elimination of wastes, is called upon promptly. More blood goes to the skin to get rid of excess heat. Even the gastrointestinal tract and the kidneys participate in an endurance exercise, not by more activity, but rather by less. At the cellular level, in almost all tissues of the body hundreds of enzymes increase their activity. This muscle energy support system involves the *whole* body.

The system can also be activated by the mind. Because of real or imaginary threats, our mind can cause an emotional disturbance in us that influences the muscle metabolism support system. The mind's stimulus originally was meant to prepare the body systems for sudden muscle work. Athletes, preparing for competition, feel the psychological stress and put it to use to make them ready. But for most sedentary people, psychological stress without muscle work can cause chronic maladjustment in the function of many different but mutually dependent body organs. Accordingly, the best time for us nonathletes to engage in physical activity is during or immediately after an emotional upset.

Our body is built for continual rhythmic sustained muscle activity. The potential capability of a newborn baby to develop an efficient muscle energy support system, *i.e.,* heart, lungs, blood vessels, endocrine glands, etc., depends on the intensity of activity that these organs will daily be called upon to provide. That potential can be developed only by increased physical activity aimed at endurance.

Our muscle energy support system was not built by nature for sedentary living or for a resting body. A healthy person, even someone over sixty-five years old, can maintain energy production at five to ten times the level needed when resting. An athlete of endurance events can sustain up to twenty times his basal metabolic rate. Why would we have this enormous capacity if it were not needed?

We cannot train our lungs, heart, and the other vital body organs in any other way than by voluntarily making our muscles need their services; without use the muscles become weak. We all have observed how weak our body feels after even a week's bedrest. Our heart must feel the same way if it has been resting due to our sedentary living habits.

AGING AND EXERCISE

Aging seems to have the same effect on the capacity of our vital organs as lack of exercise has at any age. The diminution of physiological capacities because of aging proceeds at a slower pace but is similar to the condition of a top athlete when there is a break in his training. The whole system deteriorates to the point where even our metabolism while at rest requires the system to work harder.

We tend to think of our age chronologically, but our chronological age does not represent our performance age. People of the same chronological age do not each perform a given task the same way.

If our chronological age is, say, seventy years but we have exercised our muscles and energy support system so that our performance is above the average performance of seventy-year-old people, our *performance age* is younger. The performance of our body, based on the performances of its vital functional parts, reveals our true age. *We can slow down the aging process if we keep our body and its parts functionally efficient.*

There is a definite health advantage in retarding the decline of physiological performance in advancing age. A leading authority on the biology of aging recently said, "The causes of death in the older age brackets really represent our increased vulnerability to disease. This increased vulnerability in the older age groups occurs because, as our normal physiological functions decline with age, we are less capable of dealing with diseases than we were when we were younger. Vulnerability to disease increases with age because of the slow physiological losses that normally occur within us over time. The disease causes of death therefore are simply superimposed or overlaid on top of the normal losses that we suffer in most of our bodily systems as time passes."

It seems to be rather generally agreed that of the two main aging phenomena, decline in "normal" physiological functions and the development of chronic diseases, the function decline occurs first in time. However, if we could eliminate cardiovascular disease, the prime cause of death for people sixty-five and older, we could add approximately eleven years to life expectancy even though we might not affect the functional decline. In addition, by postponing the physiological decline, we might gain another important benefit: a more energetic, productive, and independent old age.

The basic underlying danger in starting suddenly to exercise after years of sedentary living is the inability of the energy support systems to respond so abruptly. If an organ in the support system such as the heart has not been used except at a resting stage, and has imperceptibly deteriorated and possibly become prey to a disease such as atherosclerosis, it might fail in the attempt to supply the needs of the exercising muscles. The organ can function well when the body is relatively sedentary; its weakness is not revealed until the first attempt to exercise.

THE EXERCISE STRESS TEST

It is *imperative* that this first attempt to exercise, after a period of sedentary living, take place in a physician's office. This is where the capacity of the energy support systems will be measured by an exercise stress test.

In an exercise stress test, your muscle work is gradually increased in known increments and through standardized procedures. The level of muscle metabolism is raised to the point where all organs in the support system (heart, lungs, etc.) function at maximum capacity without internal damage. In this way a safe range of responses to exercise is established. Utilizing exercise test results, a qualified exercise expert can develop your personal exercise program.

The exercise expert will also advise you to forget the traditional notion of exercise as competition. The program should be recreational and an enhancement to health. The only opponent you should allow yourself, in reality or imagination, is the aging process itself. The aging process is a good opponent to play against because it can best be defeated by a cautious and gradual playing strategy. The slow and cautious strategy is appropriate not only to avoid sudden unexpected reactions in the muscle energy support organs, but also to avoid excessive strain in the "rusty" locomotive organs. Every adult suddenly starting to exercise will experience soreness in muscles and joints. These signs are harmless and will eventually disappear, but only if the exercise program is appropriate for the individual.

Remember, getting older does not change the fact that our bodies require nourishment and exercise, just as they did when we were younger. We need them in different ways, however, and our present and future health depends on our willingness to approach physical exercise especially as a competition against aging. The rewards of such competition will be better mental and physical health, and more enjoyment of the later years.

08/15 23:41 0339 TAPE11 VER-02 BY-RFM DEPTH-087.0" PAGE- PUB-ADV

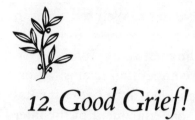

12. Good Grief!

Ralph S. Carpenter, S.T.M.

GOOD GRIEF! A contradiction of terms? What's good about grief? Probably a great deal, although that seems to be a paradox. In one way the phrase reflects our ambivalent feelings toward the expression of grief, yet at the same time it is a perfect choice to indicate the role grief plays in handling our losses.

What *is* good about grief? We must learn to look upon grief as a natural consequence of loss, but more than that, as a means through which we learn ultimately to accept the loss.

Grief is a universal experience of human beings, but it is little understood by most of us. Religious belief and practice can help us to cope with grief. However, faith will not help us if we insist that religious persons do not grieve, and that religion advocates a stoical disregard of natural human emotions, as many seem to feel it does. Some may even quote two words from the New Testament, "grieve not . . ." (I Thess. 4:13).

We tend to think of the nongriever as a brave person, and perhaps recall especially the image of Jacqueline Kennedy during that horrible weekend in November, 1963. We should have coupled our admiration for her outward calm with a recognition that her stoic attitude in the face of her calamity was probably not helpful to her, nor should it have been expected of her.

Genuinely religious persons *do* grieve. That pithy phrase in the New Testament, "Jesus wept" (John 11:35), is an indication that Jesus himself felt grief and responded to it in a very human way. The phrase "grieve not" is in fact incompletely quoted. The whole verse is, "grieve not as others do *who have no hope.*" Rev. Granger Westberg has suggested that we put a comma in this verse, and tack on a phrase, so that the verse will read, "grieve not as those who have no hope, but for goodness sake, grieve, when you have something worth grieving about!" Grief is a natural human experience, and we must not permit unrealistic and distorted religious views to hinder our capacity to cope with grief. "To say a person is deeply religious" states Westberg, "and therefore does not have to face grief situations is ridiculous. Not only is it totally unrealistic, but it is also incompatible with the whole Christian message."

Grief is not only a natural experience. It is also an inevitable experience. I refer not simply to the fact that most of us experience the loss of a loved one, but also because grief is experienced *whenever* we have a major loss. The human organism, as it develops, incorporates into its sphere of meaning the objects and persons that surround it. The pain that results from cutting one of these significant objects or persons out of our emotional constellation is what we call grief. Perhaps the person under whom you have worked happily for many years suddenly dies or is transferred, and the new man is hard to work for. Your reaction to this kind of situation may be described as a form of grief. Someone has described physical birth as our first grief experience. From then on grief extends through the various experiences of life.

Dr. Erich Lindemann of the Harvard Medical School published an article over thirty years ago that opened the eyes of many on the subject of grief reactions. He pointed to several diseases, which he called "a group of psychosomatic conditions," and which are often associated with grief experiences. In particular he pointed to ulcerative colitis, rheumatoid arthritis, and asthma. "Extensive studies in ulcerative colitis," said Dr. Lindemann, "have produced evidence that thirty-three out of forty-one patients with ulcerative colitis developed their disease in close time relationship to the loss of an important person. . . . Two of the patients developed bloody diarrhea at funerals. In the others it developed within a few weeks after the loss. The course of the ulcerative colitis was strikingly benefited when this grief reaction was resolved by psychiatric technique."

THE STAGES OF GRIEF

What then can one normally expect in the face of significant loss? We should be careful to note that I am not referring to an abnormal condition. Rather, I'm talking about the road the majority of human beings must travel in order to get back into the mainstream of life. The stages of grief were first described in Dr. Lindemann's classic article on the subject, and it is to him that I am mostly indebted at this point. As we talk about the stages of grief, we should remember that not every person goes through each stage, nor does a person necessarily go through them in the order I describe. At the conclusion of the process, however, we are likely to have gone through most of these stages in one way or another.

PHYSICAL DISTRESS. The first aspect is the presence of physical distress. For example, a marked tendency to sigh, or complain about lack of strength and exhaustion. Some common expressions we hear: "It is almost impossible to climb the stairway"; "Everything I lift seems so heavy"; "The slightest effort makes me feel exhausted." Other signs of physical distress include digestive complaints. "The food tastes like sand"; "I have no appetite at all." Or, "I stuff the food down because I have to eat."

"SEEING" THE DECEASED. A second aspect of grief is preoccupation with an image of the deceased. A patient in Dr. Lindemann's study who lost his daughter in the dreadful Coconut Grove night club fire of some years back, "visualized his girl in the telephone booth calling for him, and was much troubled by the loudness with which his name was called by her, and was so vividly preoccupied with the scene that he became oblivious to his surroundings." A young navy pilot, also in Dr. Lindemann's study, "lost a close friend; he remained a vivid part of his imagery, not in terms of religious survival, but in terms of an imaginary companion. He ate with him and talked over plans with him, for instance, discussing with him his plan to join the Air Corps." Some persons who experience this intense preoccupation with the image of their lost friend or relative are quite concerned with this. They may panic as they wonder whether they are losing their sanity. However, experiences like this are frequent, and you need not feel that you are having a unique experience when feelings like this occur.

GUILT. Even more common, however, are guilt feelings as an aspect of grief: *"If only* I had taken him to the hospital sooner than I did"; *"If only* I hadn't said what I did"; *"If only* we had taken that trip we had promised each other for so long." And so on, and so forth. The "if only" statements and feelings are extremely common, whether the grief is associated with the death of a loved one, or other significant losses such as divorce or being fired from your job. A common tack taken by friends and relatives is to see or at least sense the lack of reality implied in these guilt feelings, and to attempt to talk the bereaved out of them. How often we say, "Jane, you couldn't possibly have known how sick he was." Or, "But you were planning to take that trip this summer, and you had no possible way of knowing this would happen." Or, "You did the best you could on your job, trying to hold it, but you could not foresee the changes that led to your termination." These are well-intended remarks from friends and relatives, and usually true to the facts. In fact, she didn't know her husband was gravely ill. In fact, the trip was planned for this summer, without taking into account this sudden change of circumstances.

Nevertheless, despite good intentions and obvious truth, this kind of simple explanation does not help the bereaved. It does not take into account the guilt a person honestly feels. It is axiomatic in most counseling that you cannot solve problems by explaining them away. Mature religious faith that stresses appropriate and realistic forgiveness can be genuinely helpful to persons in this stage of the grief process, although even here the matter of appropriate timing is of critical importance. What you as a friend can provide is *active listening*—far more helpful than superficial reassurances.

RESENTMENT AND HOSTILITY. The bereaved may have feelings of resentment and hostility, which are often experienced in grief situations. According to Lindemann, "There may be a tendency to respond with irritability and anger, or a wish not to be bothered by others at a time when friends and relatives make a special effort to keep up friendly relationships." Sometimes the hostility takes the form of critical attitudes toward anyone associated with the deceased. The doctor is criticized because he operated, or because he did not. The pastor is criticized because his visits were cheerily oblivious to the serious reality of the situation, or because they were too sternly insistent on facing up to the realities obvious to everyone. Scarcely anyone can seem to please the bereaved.

The person who has such feelings finds them extremely difficult to understand, and wonders if he is losing his mind. We should recognize that ambivalent feelings of love and hate are a part of every close human relationship. While I would not want to be placed in the position of encouraging expressions of hostility, except for special purposes, we can, I think, begin to accept them as a normal part of life. This acceptance will help us to get over some of the difficult lumps that may block our growth as persons.

CHANGE IN BEHAVIOR. Fifth and last in this list of characteristic responses to grief is loss of customary patterns of conduct. As Dr. Lindemann observes, "There is no retardation of action and speech; quite to the contrary, there is a push of speech, especially when talking about the deceased. There is restlessness, inability to sit still, moving about in an aimless fashion, continually searching for something to do. There is, however, at the same time, a painful lack of capacity to initiate and maintain organized patterns of activity. What is done is done with lack of zest, as though one were going through the motions. The bereaved clings to the daily routine of prescribed activities, but these do not proceed in the automatic, self-sustaining fashion which characterizes normal work, but have to be carried on with effort, as though each fragment of the activity became a special task. The bereaved is surprised to find how large a part of his customary activity was done in some meaningful relationship to the deceased and has now lost its significance. Especially the habits of social interaction—meeting friends, making conversation, sharing enterprises with others— seem to have been lost. This loss leads to a strong dependency on anyone who will stimulate the bereaved to activity and serve as the initiating agent."

Thus far I have described characteristic grief responses. Unless our understanding leads to practical ends, there would seem to be little reason for merely describing grief or any other dynamic of our experience. Hence, I shall now focus on the healing of grief. I cannot in this brief chapter describe the entire process of grief work, as the healing process is called, but I can highlight certain features.

THE HEALING OF GRIEF

I believe that today we can begin to discuss death as an aspect of our life experience. While open discussion is not a panacea, there is some evidence to suggest that open discussion can break down the unnecessary and unreasonable mystery that surrounds this area. Someone has said that a generation ago we were prudish about sex, and the present era is prudish about death. As a culture I trust we are now ready to give up some of our reticence on this topic.

I am not suggesting that we parade the topic in an exhibitionistic fashion. An awareness of the intensely personal reactions of the bereaved at the time of death and respect for privacy require that our conversations be carried on with the utmost tact and sympathetic understanding. On the other hand, we may sometimes mistake fear of an unknown quantity for tactful silence, and our civilization is mature enough to relinquish its unnecessary fears.

Several reasons can be adduced for the more open discussion of our experiences in this regard. For one thing, there is some therapeutic value in the conversation itself. Then, too, bereavement is an inevitable part of human experience, and we can prepare ourselves and others by listening to the experiences of others. Finally, we can help persons in this situation to avoid some of the prolonged and harmful effects of unresolved grief, which research has told us can contribute to a number of human ills.

The American male is especially restricted when it comes to open expression of emotions, as David K. Switzer points out in his excellent book, *The Dynamics of Grief.*

> Our society has saddled men with a heavy burden in its expectations of the masking of emotions of sorrow and affection and tenderness. The tendency to inhibit such emotions is built into many men on an unconscious level as a result of this cultural expectation and they struggle to control them and not give expression to them too openly when they are consciously felt.

It may be well for women's liberationists to reflect that in the matter of expression of sorrow, affection, and tenderness, our society grants the female much more liberty than the male, and that is both unjust and unnecessary.

Finally, in the matter of grief work, it is impossible to escape the role of the famous triad: Faith, Hope, and Love. Love, that is, warm, close, meaningful human relationships, is obvious. "Faith," says Switzer, "is not necessarily to be thought of in a traditional sense, although for many people this may be the most meaningful framework within which to understand the other meanings in their lives." Popular definitions of faith as belief without evidence or superficial optimism that everything will turn out all right are not helpful to the bereaved. Theologian Paul Tillich's definition of faith as ultimate concern is useful. "As such," Switzer writes,

> it is seen as an act of the whole being. As act, the central force is that of present commitment, commitment to persons, causes, and meaningfulness of life, both because of the evidence for it *and* in the face of the apparent lack of it. This total commitment which affirms the meaningfulness of life and its activities and which engages the grief-stricken with other individuals and groups and causes is a necessary element in the healing of grief.

About hope, Switzer says:

> Many would want to put this [hope] in some form of traditional religious language, and would even desire to speak of the relevance of hope for the grief-stricken in terms of life after death, the continuing life of the deceased, the anticipation of reunion at some time in the future. Others find it difficult to conceive of the structure of life in this way. Nevertheless, for all persons hope can be understood as the possibility and openness toward the meaningfulness of the future which keeps faith alive and active in the present.

Grief—is it "good" or "bad"? Your own personal experience with loss will help you decide that for yourself. My belief and hope is that, in time, you can see your experiences of loss as one of many stopovers on the pilgrimage through life.

Index